Development of Me
Treatment of Opiate and
Issues for the Government and Private Sector

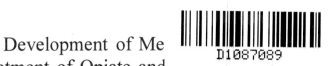

D1087089

Carolyn E. Fulco, Catharyn T. Liverman, and
Laurence E. Earley, Editors

Committee to Study Medication Development and Research
at the National Institute on Drug Abuse

Division of Biobehavioral Sciences and
Mental Disorders

INSTITUTE OF MEDICINE

NATIONAL ACADEMY PRESS
Washington, D.C. 1995

NATIONAL ACADEMY PRESS • 2101 Constitution Avenue, NW • Washington, DC 20418

NOTICE: The project that is the subject of this report was approved by the Governing Board of the National Research Council, whose members are drawn from the councils of the National Academy of Sciences, the National Academy of Engineering, and the Institute of Medicine. The members of the committee responsible for the report were chosen for their special competencies and with regard for appropriate balance.

This report has been reviewed by a group other than the authors according to procedures approved by a Report Review Committee consisting of members of the National Academy of Sciences, the National Academy of Engineering, and the Institute of Medicine.

The Institute of Medicine was chartered in 1970 by the National Academy of Sciences to enlist distinguished members of the appropriate professions in the examination of policy matters pertaining to the health of the public. In this, the Institute acts under the Academy's 1863 congressional charter responsibility to be an adviser to the federal government and its own initiative in identifying issues of medical care, research, and education. Dr. Kenneth I. Shine is president of the Institute of Medicine.

Support for this study was provided by the National Institute on Drug Abuse (contract no. N01DA-3-8000).

Library of Congress Catalog Card No. 94-80088
International Standard Book No. 0-309-05244-0

Additional copies of this report are available from:

National Academy Press
Box 285
2101 Constitution Avenue, N.W.
Washington, DC 20055

Call 800-624-6242 or 202-334-3313 (in the Washington Metropolitan Area)

B532

The serpent has been a symbol of long life, healing, and knowledge among almost all cultures and religions since the beginning of recorded history. The image adopted as a logotype by the Institute of Medicine is based on a relief carving from ancient Greece, now held by the Staalichemusseen in Berlin.

Cover: Conrad Marca-Relli, "The Blackboard," from the Eugene Fuller Memorial Collection, with permission from the Seattle Art Museum. Photo by Paul Macapia.

iii

STAFF

CAROLYN E. FULCO, Study Director
CATHARYN T. LIVERMAN, Program Officer
TERRI BARBA, Project Assistant
CONSTANCE M. PECHURA, Director, Division of Biobehavioral Sciences and Mental Disorders
ROBERT COOK-DEEGAN, Director, Division of Biobehavioral Sciences and Mental Disorders (to October, 1994)

Acknowledgments

The committee appreciates the expert support of the IOM project staff, former division director, Division of Biobehavioral Sciences and Mental Disorders (BSMD), Robert Cook-Deegan and Constance Pechura, current BSMD director, for their practical comments and guidance during the committee's deliberations. We thank study director, Carolyn Fulco for her contributions to the structure and substance of the report and in preliminary editing of this document. We are indebted to Catharyn Liverman for her excellent research skills in collecting, analyzing, and presenting a range of information, in addition to verifying all committee references; project assistant, Terri Barba for providing logistical assistance for the workshop and all committee meetings, and for overseeing report production; and Mary Ann Racin for preparing the camera-ready copy of the report.

The committee benefitted from the expertise of Miriam Davis and her input into the committee's deliberations and of Robert Talbot-Stern, consultants to the committee. The committee wishes to express its sincere appreciation to Geoffrey M. Levitt for his excellent research and expert legal advice. The committee appreciates the overall editing by Norman Grossblatt and Kate Kelly; and the assistance of Claudia Carl in guiding the report through review.

The IOM staff and the committee appreciate the thoughtful input and contribution of Charles Grudzinskas and his staff at NIDA. We are also indebted to the many representatives of federal agencies, congressional staff, academia, advocacy groups, professional organizations, and the pharmaceutical industry who shared their expertise with the committee. Those individuals are acknowledged in Appendix A.

Preface

Pharmacotherapy for the treatment of drug addiction has received far too little attention, despite the clinical success of methadone, which dates back to the 1960s. Over the last 30 years only two additional medications have been approved for the treatment of opiate addiction, naltrexone and levo-alpha-acetylmethadol (LAAM), and it is important to note that both of those medications were developed in the 1960s and early 1970s. There is no approved medication for the treatment of cocaine addiction. During the same 30 year period, serious medical and social problems have evolved as drug addiction has become a route for spreading AIDS through the sharing of contaminated needles and trading sex for drugs, multiple-drug-resistant tuberculosis has become common in immunocompromised HIV-infected drug users, an association between illicit drug use and increasing violent crime has become clear, and the medical consequences for infants of in utero exposure to cocaine has become evident.

It was in the climate of a near absence of private sector and government activity in the development of anti-addiction medications and a growing public health crisis that the Congress passed Public Law 100-690 in 1988, which established the Medications Development Division (MDD) in the National Institute on Drug Abuse (NIDA). The division began in 1990 to coordinate and encourage academic, private, and federal regulatory involvement in developing and bringing to market new medications for the treatment of drug addiction.

The ADAMHA Reorganization Act of July 1992 (Public Law 102-321) stipulated that the Department of Health and Human Services contract with the National Academy of Sciences to establish a committee of the Institute of Medicine (IOM) to examine the current environment for the development of anti-addiction medications. In response to the Congressional mandate, the Committee to Study Medication Development and Research at the National Institute on Drug Abuse was formed. The 14-member interdisciplinary IOM committee included persons with expertise in behavioral pharmacology, drug abuse treatment, neuroscience, drug development, health-care economics, clinical research, and federal regulatory law.

NIDA and IOM decided that a two-phase effort would most beneficially address the complex issues associated with the development of an anti-addiction medication. The committee was charged to

- Determine the extent to which current scientific knowledge limits the development of pharmacological treatments for drug addiction,
- Review the background and progress of the NIDA MDD since its inception in 1990,
- Consider the current role of the Food and Drug Administration (FDA) and other government entities in the process for approving anti-addiction medications,
- Survey the incentives and disincentives to private development of medications including government regulatory processes and the potential market for anti-addiction medications, and
- Determine the current role of the private sector in the development of medications for drug addiction.

The committee focused its attention exclusively on medications for treating opiate and cocaine addictions, because individuals with those addictions are disproportionately responsible for violent crimes and for the transmission of infectious diseases such as AIDS. The committee recognizes, however, that the two addictive drugs that are most important with respect to morbidity, mortality, and economic costs are alcohol and nicotine.

The committee formally met six times during the course of the entire study, in addition to holding a workshop, and meeting in smaller focus groups. From October 1993 through January 1994 the IOM committee met three times to examine the role of the Medications Development Division at NIDA and identify the disincentives to private sector development of anti-addiction medications specifically for the treatment of opiate and cocaine addictions. Additionally, the committee met with senior executives of pharmaceutical companies, representatives of federal agencies (the Drug Enforcement Administration, NIDA, the National Institutes of Health, and FDA), and the IOM Forum on Drug Development, as well as conducting a survey of the member companies of the Pharmaceutical Research and Manufacturers of America (formerly the Pharmaceutical Manufacturers Association), the Biotechnology Industry Organization (BIO), and the Generic Pharmaceutical Industry Association (GPIA). The committee issued its preliminary report, *Development of Anti-Addiction Medications: Issues for the Government and Private Sector,* in March 1994 which was disseminated to NIDA, ONDCP, various Congressional committees, other interested parties, and was the subject of a Senate Judiciary Committee hearing on April 19, 1994.

The committee held its final three meetings, from April 1994 through September 1994. During the second phase of its work, the committee:

- provided a more detailed examination of the issues identified in the preliminary report regarding disincentives to private sector development of anti-addiction medications,
- further assessed the market environment for developing those medications, and
- recommended policy and legislative solutions for overcoming the obstacles and disincentives for the development of anti-addiction medications.

The committee heard from a wide range of experts at their June 13, 1994 Workshop on Policies to Stimulate Private Sector Development of Anti-Addiction Medications; sessions focused on market issues, treatment financing, federal and state regulations regarding substance abuse research and treatment, and education and training (see Appendix F for workshop agenda and participant list). This report combines the two phases of the committee's work; the organization and content of the report are outlined in the Note to the Reader.

The committee, recognizing the medical consequences and socioeconomic problems associated with drug abuse and the dire need for development of anti-addiction medications, yet fully aware of the major disincentives to the industry, grappled with the issue of providing extraordinary incentives to the pharmaceutical industry. Several ideas were discussed at length, including those that were presented at the workshop. These included, granting a patent-extension on some other product marketed by a pharmaceutical company that develops an approved anti-addiction medication; removing the potential for price controls; advance special purchase of an anti-addiction medication; and/or creating a prize or bounty to the first few companies that produce an approved anti-addiction medication. Although, the committee could not adequately envision the implementation of those extraordinary incentives and did not reach a consensus to make specific recommendations on those issues, a majority of the committee agreed that certain of the incentives regarded as extraordinary should be deliberated by policymakers. Thus, in the final chapter of the report, two of those issues, which had support from a majority of the committee members, are presented, not as recommendations, but as approaches for further consideration.

As the committee worked throughout the year on the issue of developing anti-addiction medications, it become obvious that such medications could have enormous benefit and positive impact not only on the lives of drug-dependent individuals but on many aspects of American society. The committee is aware of recent studies which note that every dollar spent on drug treatment is worth seven dollars spent on law-enforcement efforts, clearly demonstrating the cost-effectiveness of treatment. Yet, pharmacotherapy, as an effective and viable adjunct to other treatment modalities, has received far too little attention from the research community, the pharmaceutical industry, public health officials, and the federal government. The committee considered obstacles, large and small, that impede the development of anti-addiction medications. It is the hope of this committee that the issues discussed in this report and its recommendations well be carefully considered not only by the National Institute on Drug Abuse, but also by the Congress and the executive branch as policy options for treating drug addiction are examined and priorities are set.

Laurence E. Earley
Committee Chair

Note to the Reader

This report is the result of a two-phase study as explained in the preface. The first phase of the work of the IOM Committee to Study Medication Development and Research at NIDA resulted in the desk-top published report, *Development of Anti-Addiction Medications: Issues for the Government and Private Sector.* That preliminary report was published in March 1994 and was available through the IOM Division of Biobehavioral Sciences and Mental Disorders. It was the intent of the Institute of Medicine to publish the report through the National Academy Press after both phases of the study had been completed; this report incorporates both phases of the committee's work. The chapters in this, the final report, have been reorganized from the preliminary report as follows:

- A preface to the final edition
- An executive summary
- Chapters 1–3, unchanged
- Chapters 4–6, new text from the second phase of the committee's work
- Chapter 7, the text from Chapter 4 of the preliminary report (originally entitled "The Interaction of Federal Regulatory Agencies and the Private Sector")
- Chapter 8, new text from the second phase of the committee's work
- Chapter 9, incorporates Chapter 5 of the preliminary report with additional text and recommendations

Minor changes were made in Chapters 1–3 and 7 to update prevalence statistics, add cross-references, and incorporate the erratum to the preliminary report.

Contents

APPENDIXES

Tables, Figures, and Boxes

TABLES

FIGURES

BOXES

Development of Medications for the Treatment of Opiate and Cocaine Addictions: Issues for the Government and Private Sector

Executive Summary

Pharmacotherapy for the treatment of drug addiction[1] has received far too little attention, despite the clinical success of methadone, which dates back to the 1960s. Over the last 30 years, only two additional medications have been approved for the treatment of opiate addiction—naltrexone and levo-alpha-acetylmethadol (LAAM)—and it is important to note that both those medications were developed in the 1960s and early 1970s. There is still no approved medication for the treatment of cocaine addiction. During the same 30 year period, however, serious medical and social problems have evolved as drug addiction has become a route for spreading the acquired immune deficiency syndrome (AIDS) through the sharing of contaminated needles and the trading of sex for drugs; multiple-drug-resistant tuberculosis has become common in immunocompromised, human immunodeficiency virus (HIV) infected drug-dependent individuals; an association between illicit drug use and increasing violent crime has become clear; and the medical consequences for infants exposed in utero to cocaine have become evident (Chapter 1). It is for those reasons and others (Chapter 3) that the committee focused its attention on medications to treat opiate and cocaine addictions, although it recognizes that the two addictive drugs that are most important with respect to morbidity, mortality, and economic costs are alcohol and nicotine.

---

[1]Drug addiction is defined as the compulsive use of a drug despite adverse consequences. This report focuses on opiate and cocaine addictions and does not address alcohol and nicotine addictions.

Given the magnitude of the illicit-drug-use problem (there are an estimated 0.5–1 million heroin-dependent individuals and 2.1 million cocaine-dependent individuals) and its economic and public-health consequences, addressing the issue requires a dedicated effort not only to develop pharmacotherapies but also to foster prevention, education, and the use of other treatment approaches. Yet, pharmacotherapy, as a viable adjunct to other treatment modalities, has not received widespread support from the federal government, nor has the private sector been active in developing anti-addiction medications.

It was in this climate of a near absence of private-sector and government activity in the development of anti-addiction medications that Congress established the Medications Development Division (MDD) in the National Institute on Drug Abuse (NIDA). The division began in 1990 to coordinate and encourage academic, private, and federal regulatory involvement in developing and bringing to market new medications for the treatment of drug addiction. In 1992, the Congress stipulated in the Alcohol, Drug Abuse, and Mental Health Administration (ADAMHA) Reorganization Act (P.L. 102-321) that the Department of Health and Human Services contract with the National Academy of Sciences to establish a committee in the Institute of Medicine (IOM) to examine the current conditions for the development of anti-addiction medications. This report by the IOM Committee to Study Medication Development and Research at the National Institute on Drug Abuse responds to the Congressional mandate by examining the progress of NIDA's Medications Development Division and exploring the scientific, marketplace, regulatory, and other factors that adversely affect the development of anti-addiction medications. The committee met with representatives of the IOM Drug Forum, the pharmaceutical industry, and federal agencies—NIDA, the Food and Drug Administration (FDA), and the Drug Enforcement Administration (DEA)—conducted a survey of the pharmaceutical industry, and sponsored a Workshop on Policies to Stimulate Private Sector Development of Anti-Addiction Medications.

As a result of the committee's deliberations, meetings, and workshop, it became evident that the major disincentives to pharmaceutical R&D for anti-addiction medications include: an inadequate science base on addiction and the prevention of relapse (especially for cocaine); an uncertain market environment which includes such issues as: treatment financing, lack of trained specialists for the treatment of drug addiction, federal and state regulations, market size, pricing issues, societal stigma, liability issues, difficulties in conducting clinical research; and a lack of sustained federal leadership.

STATE OF THE SCIENTIFIC KNOWLEDGE ON ADDICTION

The initiating event leading to drug addiction is the administration of an agent, such as heroin or cocaine, to obtain a pleasurable effect. Addiction is characterized as the compulsive use of a drug despite adverse consequences. Key problems in addiction are how to prevent the onset of compulsive drug use and how to prevent relapse and the craving that leads to relapse (Chapter 2). In the past, much medical attention has been given to treatment (detoxification) for the symptoms of acute abstinence. Yet, knowledge about the pathophysiology of the syndromes of protracted abstinence and conditioned withdrawal or relapse is still rudimentary and presents an important challenge to development of anti-addiction medications.

Since the 1960s, it has become clear that the effects of opiate drugs are mediated through interaction with opioid receptors and interference with actions at those receptors presents a rational strategy for developing medications for opiate addiction. The mechanism of cocaine addiction is not well characterized, however, it is understood that the major pharmacological effect of cocaine is on the dopaminergic system of the brain. Unfortunately, the potential involvement of a wide range of neurotransmitter systems in cocaine's actions makes the development of a treatment medication difficult because no single target site is immediately apparent. In fact, an optimal strategy might require the use of several drugs that have different mechanisms of action.

In response to the absence of a well-defined mechanism of action or a compound for the treatment of cocaine addiction, MDD has developed the Cocaine Treatment Discovery Program (CTDP) to screen candidate compounds through a tiered strategy that uses both in vitro biochemical assays and in vivo behavioral tests. However, several factors limit the effectiveness of the screening protocols and their predictive value in humans, including the lack of knowledge of the mechanism of cocaine addiction; the lack of animal models for addiction, craving, and relapse; and the small number of compounds supplied to NIDA for screening. In its report, the committee makes several specific recommendations to MDD regarding the CTDP program.

Because the state of scientific knowledge of addiction is rudimentary, the committee believes that it is imperative to foster NIDA's basic-research efforts in the mechanism of cocaine addiction and in the molecular, cellular, and behavioral bases of chronic drug effects and the genetics of vulnerability to addiction. There is also a need for basic research to develop laboratory models of behavioral characteristics of the addictive process. The committee strongly believes that unless basic research is supported at an appropriate funding level, it will be difficult to make the necessary progress in the scientific knowledge base. The lack of such knowledge would continue to hamper the private sector and MDD in the development of a medication.

In relation specifically to MDD, the committee recommends two mechanisms to address the critical issue of supporting basic science:

The committee recommends that MDD be given a high priority for funding. Although MDD was authorized at $95 million in FY 1994, its appropriation of $40 million was considerably short of its authorization and is far below what is needed for research and development.

The committee is aware, however, of the budget constraints on the institutes of the National Institutes of Health (NIH); as a possible mechanism for increased support, the committee suggests the use of funds from the Special Forfeiture Fund in the Office of National Drug Control Policy (ONDCP).[2] Utilizing a portion of those funds for basic research not only would provide additional money to MDD, but would demonstrate executive-branch support.

The committee recommends that NIDA designate national drug abuse research centers, subject to congressional appropriations, as described in the ADAMHA Reorganization Act [P.L. 102-321, Section 464N (a)], "for the purpose of interdisciplinary research relating to drug abuse and other biomedical, behavioral, and social issues related to drug abuse." Those centers would be engaged in and would coordinate all aspects of drug-abuse research, treatment, and education.

The paucity of basic knowledge is best approached through a coordinated effort, and the committee intends that such centers serve as focal points for all

---

[2]The ONDCP Special Forfeiture Fund results from the transfer of money from the Federal Asset Forfeiture Fund (described below). In FY 1990, the Federal Asset Forfeiture Fund transferred $117 million to federal law-enforcement agencies. Deposits of $17 million were also made to the Special Forfeiture Fund to supplement ONDCP program resources and of $115 million to support Federal prison construction. The use of the Special Forfeiture Fund is at the discretion of the director of ONDCP.

The Federal Asset Forfeiture Fund is a sum of money resulting from the sale of assets used in criminal activity that have been seized by the government. In 1990, DEA seized assets valued at more than $1 billion. About two-fifths of the assets seized by DEA was currency valued at almost $364 million. In addition, DEA seized $346 million worth of real property, 5,674 vehicles worth over $60 million, 187 vessels valued at over $16 million, and 51 airplanes worth over $25 million. Almost two-thirds of DEA's seizures during 1990 resulted from cocaine investigations. DEA seizures that were ultimately forfeited are valued at more than $427 million in 1990.

aspects of drug-abuse research and their designation would have the added benefit of encouraging new investigators to enter the field; the centers would also serve as sites for clinical trials and for training clinicians. With the designation of such centers, the committee believes, progress will be made in basic and clinical research on the treatment of drug addiction (Chapter 2).

NIDA'S MEDICATIONS DEVELOPMENT DIVISION

In recognition of the need to stimulate the availability of medications to treat drug addiction, the Anti-Drug Abuse Act of 1988 (P.L. 100-690) authorized funds for a drug discovery and development program in NIDA. Beginning with an appropriation of $8 million in 1988, NIDA launched a Medications Development Program in its Division of Preclinical Research. Building on this program, NIDA formally established the Medications Development Division in 1990. The primary strategy adopted by MDD is to work with industry to perform the research and development necessary to secure FDA marketing approval for new medications to treat drug addiction. MDD does not operate inhouse laboratories or clinical-development programs to fulfill its mission. It manages this work through multiple external instruments, such as contracts, grants, and interagency and collaborative agreements (Chapter 3).

While the current budget of $40 million and staff of 33 full-time equivalents (FTEs) might be adequate to support the development of a small portfolio of products based on drugs that are already in use, the committee believes that they are insufficient to support basic research. Additionally, MDD has had difficulty in stimulating private-sector interest, in acquiring industry partners, and in obtaining a suitable number of compounds for screening. MDD had originally developed a screening agreement in which a compound's structure is made public after a 3-year period of confidentiality. That agreement has hindered MDD's ability to acquire compounds and affected MDD's capability to develop its screening program adequately because many companies did not want their confidential data to be made public. Thus, in 1994 MDD revised their original screening agreement and now all screening data from industry compounds will remain confidential. That change in policy should have a beneficial effect on MDD's screening program.

Although the committee commends MDD for the establishment of anti-cocaine and anti-opiate screening programs, the lack of established in vitro screening methods and validated animal models that are predictive in humans, especially for anti-cocaine medications, limits the utility of the screening program. The committee feels that there is a need for basic research to develop laboratory models of critical behavioral characteristics of the addictive process.

Improvement of such methods and models should be given a high priority for grant and contract support by MDD.

It became apparent to the committee, during its review of MDD and numerous meetings with industry representatives, that strong leadership is needed in promoting pharmacotherapy as an important component of our national strategy. Leadership must come from many sources, especially from the highest levels of the federal bureaucracy. However, an important leadership role belongs uniquely to NIDA and especially to MDD. MDD must view itself as the leader in stimulating private-sector interest in developing anti-addiction medications. The committee views this national leadership role as one of the key functions of MDD. Consequently, it should be empowered to lead, as well as to fulfill, a scientific and technical mission.

> **The committee recommends that NIDA and MDD, in determining how to improve MDD's relationship with industry, evaluate the applicability of the techniques already in use by the Developmental Therapeutics Program of the National Cancer Institute, the National Cooperative Drug Discovery Groups on Acquired Immune Deficiency Syndrome of the National Institute of Allergy and Infectious Disease, and the Anticonvulsant Drug Development Program of the National Institute of Neurological Disorders and Stroke.**

Those are all programs (Appendix E) of similar mission within NIH that have established effective working relationships among leading academic and government scientists, FDA, and individual drug companies through a combination of scientific communication, mutual technical assistance, cooperative agreements, and licenses. In the committee's view, the primary policy responsibility of MDD should be to provide such leadership as a complement to its scientific responsibilities (Chapter 3).

EFFECTIVENESS OF TREATMENT

There is strong consensus that methadone maintenance treatment is effective for the treatment of opiate addiction (IOM, 1990; OTA, 1990; Anglin and Hser, 1992; Prendergast et al., in press). Treatment is effective in reducing opiate use, criminal activity, and intravenous drug use. The evidence of treatment effectiveness is not as strong for cocaine treatment, yet there is an accumulating body of research pointing to the effectiveness of psychosocial treatment modalities. As yet, there is not a pharmacologic agent for the treatment of cocaine addiction or a medication to reduce cocaine craving.

Treatments for opiate and cocaine addiction are cost-effective (Chapter 4). When the cost of opiate and cocaine treatment is compared to the benefits in reduced crime, the result is unambiguous: every dollar invested in treatment yields at least two and up to four dollars, and sometimes more, in societal benefits (Gerstein et al., 1994). Treatment also averts other health care costs. In short, current treatments for opiate and cocaine addiction, while variable in nature and cost, are both effective and cost-effective. Clearly the federal government should make every effort to expand the treatment capabilities of the states. New medications, especially for cocaine addiction, do hold the potential to reduce some of the need for counseling, which forms the largest share of treatment charges. With lower overall treatment costs, treatment can prove to become even more cost-effective.

The committee strongly recommends expanding the treatment capabilities of the states for opiate- and cocaine-dependent individuals to ensure that all those seeking treatment obtain it without delay. The recommendation may be implemented by:

- **Providing additional money to increase treatment in states where there are waiting lists.**
- **Shifting money from supply control programs to treatment programs.**

TREATMENT FINANCING

The financing[3] of treatment is often cited by the pharmaceutical industry as yet another deterrent to the development of anti-addiction medications (Chapter 5). Prominent reasons are the fact that so few patients have private insurance and there is a concomitant need to rely on direct public subsidy to pay for their treatment (IOM Workshop, June 13, 1994).

The annual payments for methadone maintenance treatment are estimated at $480 million in FY 1993. There are an estimated 117,000 patients for whom annual expenditures are about $4,100 each. Currently the financing of methadone treatment is deeply dependent on the public sector, primarily in the form of federal block grants and state alcohol and drug agency funds. Despite the sizeable public role in financing, neither state agencies or the federal government have

---

[3]Financing is generally defined as the payment or reimbursement for the cost of treatment made by private insurance, Medicaid, the patients themselves, or other sources. Financing is important to pharmaceutical investment because it has a critical effect treatment supply and the demand of treatment (Rogowski, 1993).

consolidated their potential market leverage to secure discounts on large volume pharmaceutical purchases. Private insurance payment is almost insignificant. Patients are willing to pay their share, but were treatment to become more costly, patients are not likely to have the resources to absorb increased costs.

State financing has been and is expected to be a major impediment to the sale of LAAM, according to both BioDevelopment and clinic operators. State financing practices can be so rigid that they effectively block the introduction and adoption of a new medication. The flow of funds to clinics is dictated by the policies and regulations of two separate state agencies: the state alcohol and drug agency, which administers state funds and federal block grants, and the state Medicaid agency, which administers state and federal Medicaid dollars. There is widespread variation in funding practices (IOM, 1995), but either state agency can erect financial barriers to the adoption of a new medication. New York set a flat daily or weekly fee per patient (which usually includes all services without specifying the amount for medication and dispensing), and other states have set a flat fee for a "dosing visit," the dispensing of one dose of medication. California, authorizes ceilings on the number of publicly funded patients that can be treated at each clinic (Goldstein, 1989). Under these funding practices, LAAM is at a disadvantage because it is more expensive than methadone, the medication for which reimbursement rates have been structured over the past 20 years. To obtain better reimbursement, clinics must petition the appropriate agency for more favorable rates.

Financing and regulatory obstacles are contributing to the stalled market penetration of LAAM. LAAM's higher price may have exacerbated the problem, but the rigidity of the financing and regulatory structure antedates its introduction. This is unfortunate as LAAM is potentially more effective therapeutically. Even one of LAAM's selling points for public health—the prospect of increasing clinic patient loads—has become a disincentive for state alcohol and drug authorities struggling to find additional funding not just for LAAM, but for the higher costs of counseling and comprehensive treatment for possibly more patients. If BioDevelopment Corporation succeeds in securing adequate financing, that will serve as an incentive to other pharmaceutical companies. If not, the future for other opiate medications does not appear encouraging. Therefore, the committee strongly urges state and federal agencies to work together, not only to provide an incentive to pharmaceutical companies, but in the interest of public health, to facilitate the availability of newly approved anti-addiction medications. Possible mechanisms that the states and federal government might consider include requiring all Substance Abuse Block Grant recipients to offer those medications to patients and assuring appropriate financing of new medications by state alcohol and drug agencies and their counterpart Medicaid agencies. Those actions would have the additional benefit of providing a strong signal to pharmaceutical companies demonstrating state and federal commitment to the development of anti-addiction medications (Chapter 5).

TRAINING AND EDUCATION

Although the limited availability of scientists and clinicians specializing in drug abuse research and treatment has direct consequences for the delivery of health care services and research on new treatments, it has a less obvious, but equally important, effect on pharmaceutical R&D investment. Pharmaceutical companies traditionally market their products to health care professionals and promote their products through personal visits by sales representatives, through journal and mail advertising, and through support of scientific symposia and continuing medical education. Pharmaceutical companies distribute their products through hospital and community pharmacies, pharmacy chains, and distributors. To the extent that the treatment of drug dependence is often delivered outside that system by specialized clinics (e.g., narcotic treatment programs, typically with part-time physicians and limited marketing opportunities for pharmaceutical companies), and to the extent that drug abuse treatment involves many fields of medicine (e.g., family practice, internal medicine, psychiatry), pharmaceutical companies see greater difficulty in marketing anti-addiction medications than in marketing other products. Pharmaceutical firms also rely on academic clinical investigators and practicing clinicians to advise them on drug development issues such as current therapeutic trends, the role of drugs in the overall treatment strategy, unmet medical needs, indications to be evaluated, clinical trial design, and appropriate therapeutic endpoints.

The committee believes that a long-term national effort is needed to strengthen the substance abuse education and training of both specialists and primary care physicians. That effort will strengthen the infrastructure needed for research and treatment and will encourage pharmaceutical investment in this field (Chapter 6).

The committee recommends that the federal government increase its efforts to attract researchers and clinicians to the field of drug addiction treatment. That may be accomplished by implementing one or all of the following options:

- **NIDA's training budget could be increased, but not at the expense of their research programs. Requests from NIDA for large increases in its training budget have not been filled in FY 1993 or FY 1994, and NIDA has received a lower percentage of training funds than several other institutes. Increasing NIDA's training** budget such that it will enable NIDA to offer fellowships that are competitive with private sector salaries, and therefore, more attractive to potential candidates would "jump-start" the expansion of the field of drug addiction treatment and research; it could have nationwide impact by increasing the numbers of scientists and physicians recruited, trained, and working in the field of drug addiction.

•   An educational loan repayment program in return for work in drug abuse-related clinical research could attract young physicians with substantial educational debt into careers as clinical investigators.
•   Mid-career programs could be developed to encourage a cadre of practicing physicians and scientists to enter the field of drug addiction treatment and research.

The committee recommends an increased emphasis on drug abuse education throughout medical school and primary care residency programs. To accomplish this, the following could be implemented:

•   Drug abuse education could follow a systematic, integrated approach to coordinate the curriculum across specialty departments.
•   Training institutions could develop affiliations with community-based treatment centers, where feasible, to provide student access to multiple treatment settings.
•   The National Board of Medical Examiners[4] and the primary care specialty boards of the American Board of Medical Specialties (ABMS) could pay increased attention to drug abuse issues, skills, and knowledge on their examinations for certification.
•   Faculty development programs could receive increased federal support. The Center for Substance Abuse Prevention's Faculty Development Program which trains medical school faculty members to serve as role models, educators, and mentors in the field of drug abuse research and treatment is a good model.

The committee recommends that comprehensive drug abuse centers be developed to engage in and coordinate all aspects of drug-abuse research, treatment, and education. Further, the committee recom-

---

[4]The National Board of Medical Examiners prepares and administers to medical students a two-part examination that is accepted by individual states as part of licensing.

mends that NIDA and the Substance Abuse and Mental Health Services Administration (SAMHSA) work together to coordinate the effective and efficient use of existing centers by adding, where feasible, research, training, and/or treatment components.

FEDERAL REGULATORY ISSUES

Food and Drug Administration

Clinical testing and market approval of any new medication requires compliance with the regulatory requirements of FDA. In recent years, the traditional approval process has undergone changes designed to expedite FDA review and to expand the use of experimental treatments under some circumstances. The recent changes to the traditional drug-approval process might provide additional opportunities for encouraging and expediting the development of anti-addiction medications. Of particular importance are three initiatives intended to expedite the availability of drugs to treat serious and life-threatening diseases for which no adequate therapeutic alternatives exist (Chapter 7). First, under the treatment-IND (investigational new drug) regulations, FDA may approve the distribution of an investigational drug outside the context of controlled clinical trials to treat patients with serious or immediately life-threatening diseases for which no comparable or satisfactory alternative therapy is available. A second mechanism, known as parallel track, also extends the availability of investigational drugs. Under parallel track, "promising" investigational agents may be provided to patients who are not able to take standard therapy or for whom standard therapy is no longer effective and who are not able to participate in clinical trials. The third important development is FDA's accelerated-approval-program. Adopted in its final form in December 1992, accelerated approval is available for drugs that offer "meaningful therapeutic benefit compared to existing treatment" for serious or life-threatening illnesses. As an incentive to the pharmaceutical industry and because drug addiction should qualify as a serious and life-threatening disease,

The committee recommends that FDA make the treatment-IND route, the parallel-track mechanism, and accelerated approval available for anti-addiction medications.

Drug Enforcement Administration

FDA's approval of an anti-addiction drug does not necessarily end the regulatory requirements for marketing the drug. If the drug is a narcotic itself or is subject to abuse, as are methadone or LAAM, it is subject to regulation as a controlled substance by DEA. Such regulations affect the ability to conduct clinical research, require extensive paperwork and inspection, and delay marketing of a medication. The committee examined current DEA regulations that act as disincentives to industry, and made recommendations to reduce those disincentives (Chapter 7). For example, in calculating the review period for controlled substances, FDA does not count the time lost after approval of an NDA (new drug application) through scheduling by DEA. That time is unrecoverable by the manufacturer and cited as a reason for lack of interest in developing medications that might be controlled (scheduled) substances.

The committee recommends that DEA review time be counted as part of the regulatory process for purposes of patent term extension for controlled substances.[5]

To accomplish this, any of the following three options could be implemented:

•   **Amend the Drug Price Competition and Patent Term Restoration Act (DPC-PTR).**
•   **Concurrent DEA scheduling and FDA approval, in the final stages of drug review.**
•   **Unilateral FDA reversion to its earlier policy of issuing NDA "approvable" letters for drugs proposed for scheduling.**

Furthermore, the Controlled Substances Act (CSA) and DEA's regulations require that persons conducting clinical research with any controlled substance register with DEA, keep specific kinds of records, and make periodic reports to

---

[5]In the mid-1980s, FDA routinely issued NDA "approvable" letters for drugs proposed for scheduling. In 1986, FDA changed its policy regarding NDA approvals for drugs pending scheduling and issued final "approval" letters with the addition of a statement that the drug could not be marketed until it was scheduled by DEA. The result was that the "clock" measuring time before patent expiration, for DPC-PTR Act purposes, was started, even though the drug was not able to be marketed. Under current FDA policy, issuance of a final approval letter seems to permit sale under the Food, Drug and Cosmetic Act without restriction, and no provision of the Controlled Substances Act applies to a drug that is not controlled under that Act.

DEA. In addition, DEA requires that protocols for research with Schedule I controlled substances be submitted to it for approval and requires researchers using Schedule I substances to identify in their registration applications the extent to which the research will also involve manufacture or importation. The practical consequences of this dual authority over clinical research, particularly in the light of the additional complication of multiple state laws patterned after the CSA, is a clinical research environment for scheduled drugs that is extraordinarily bureaucratic from the procedural point of view and unnecessarily difficult. That is especially true given the relatively small amounts of any controlled substance used in research; the consequences of diversion to public health would be small even if the diversion was substantial. It should also be noted that even if the new drug under study is not scheduled, the comparative agent in positively controlled studies of the drug (which might well be the pivotal studies for FDA approval) could be a controlled substance like methadone; this would trigger the complex dual system of regulation noted above.

The committee recommends that action be taken to remove the adverse effects of DEA requirements, under the CSA, on clinical research investigations involving controlled substances, by holders of active FDA INDs, either by amending the CSA to exempt such investigations from applicable DEA regulations or by the alternative administrative and regulatory measures:

• The development of a Memorandum of Understanding between FDA and DEA governing the matter of dual authority over clinical research to provide exemption from DEA reporting requirements.
• DEA revision of 21 CFR 1301.33 and parallel regulations to provide that protocols, drug security, recordkeeping, production controls, reporting, and other requirements would be governed by the FDA regulations and monitored by FDA. This would require parallel changes in FDA's IND regulations.

FDA's current provisions for control and recording the disposition of controlled substances under an IND, as noted above, should be adequate to address concerns of drug security and diversion (Chapter 7).

STATE REGULATORY ISSUES

State laws and regulations also affect the discovery, development, and marketing of anti-addiction medications, especially if the medication is a controlled substance (Chapter 8). Current medications to treat opiate addiction (methadone and LAAM) are schedule II narcotics that are tightly regulated, not only under the federal CSA and the Narcotic Addict Treatment Act (NATA) but under companion state laws. There are 51 sets of laws and regulations (for each state and the District of Columbia), that are counterparts to the comprehensive federal regulatory structure for controlled substances.

State and federal controlled substances acts are designed primarily to govern the possession, use, sale, distribution, and manufacture of medications that have a potential for abuse. Most state CSAs contain regulatory mechanisms, terminology, and provisions similar to those contained in the federal CSA; although, there are significant differences between federal provisions and states' provisions and variations in statutes from one state to another (NCJA, 1991). A failure to understand the regulatory framework in each state can lead to significant delays in clinical research development, marketing and use of a new anti-addiction medication, as shown by a case study of LAAM (Chapter 8). Any perceived delay in a return on investment to a pharmaceutical company can influence the decision to develop a new anti-addiction medication. Inasmuch as this area is already perceived as a marginal business investment, the additional overlay of the state regulations and the resulting delays can further deter companies from entering this field of medications development. That could be particularly true for smaller companies that have limited regulatory resources. Smaller companies may have an additional disadvantage if they have a limited number of products, and cannot afford the time lag before realizing a return on their investment.

A case study of the state regulatory hurdles faced in the market launch of LAAM, highlights some of the problems resulting from state regulations and demonstrates that state by state acceptance of LAAM, for marketing purposes, has been necessary even after final FDA approval of LAAM and rescheduling by DEA. The regulatory areas that pose the greatest problems for LAAM are scheduling and rescheduling procedures, amendment of treatment regulations, and the approval of treatment clinics. As illustrated by LAAM, regulatory regimes that were created with the intention of controlling abuse of illicit substances can prove unwieldy and counterproductive when they are applied to a therapeutic product. Of course, future anti-addiction medications might not be Schedule I or II narcotics—or even controlled substances—in which case many of the problems associated with LAAM would not occur.

While state inactivity is rescheduling can result in long delays in moving a drug from schedule I (under state Controlled Substances Acts) to schedules II to V, this situation is brought about in part by the current federal policy of interpreting "currently accepted medical use in treatment in the United States" (for purposes of scheduling under the Controlled Substances Act) as requiring NDA approval. As a consequence of this policy is that the regulatory process at the federal level is prolonged for all newly approved drugs that are controlled substances (Chapter 7); this regulatory delay can become years when the rescheduling process requires both state and federal action and cannot begin until NDA approval, e.g., LAAM. The committee believes that the public health would be best served by an interpretation of the "currently accepted medical use" clause in the Controlled Substances Act that would recognize the use in humans under an IND and permit the scheduling process to begin at the time of NDA submission. The information required for scheduling a drug is already required to be in a self-contained section of the NDA. That section could be reviewed on a fast-track basis by FDA, and a scheduling recommendation could be sent to DEA well ahead of NDA approval. Scheduling could be done contingent upon final FDA approval. That approach would permit states to reschedule schedule I drugs closer in time to final FDA approval, minimizing delays such as the one now affecting LAAM, and have no negative drug control implications. Furthermore, it would remove a significant regulatory disincentive at the federal level that affects all scheduled drugs, not just schedule I substances. The committee concludes that if the current situation continues unchanged, it will have a chilling effect on private sector investment for any medication that may potentially meet the legal definition of a narcotic.

The committee recommends that the Office of National Drug Control Policy (ONDCP) direct DEA, in consultation with FDA and NIDA, to revise its policy on determining when a drug has a currently accepted medical use in treatment so that, for new therapeutic drugs that are also controlled substances, the process of scheduling can begin as soon as possible after submission of the NDA.

The committee believes that additional steps should be taken by federal agencies within the existing system to reduce future state obstacles. The committee proposes a two-step set of actions, interim and long-term. There are two interim steps federal agencies (ONDCP, FDA, SAMHSA, NIDA, and DEA) should take under existing authorities to ameliorate the delays, complexity, and lack of uniformity at the state level.

Interim Actions

The committee recommends that federal agencies (ONDCP, NIDA, SAMHSA, FDA, and DEA) work more closely and actively with state regulatory authorities early in the drug development process

to prepare the path for new anti-addiction medications. That recommendation can be implemented as follows:

- Identification of a regulatory point of contact in each state;
- Basic information could be given to the state contact early in the drug development process (preferably no later than the submission of an NDA) about the medication, with emphasis on characteristics that would be of most interest to state regulatory authorities (diversion potential, target populations, or any special characteristics that would affect how the drug would be dispensed, such as dosing frequency). To the extent that any of the information is proprietary and confidential, the developer's permission for such disclosure would have to be obtained.
- As the medication moves closer to FDA approval, federal agencies could ensure that the necessary state regulatory processes begin immediately after approval, or, if state regulations permit, even before, such as upon the issuance of an approvable letter.
- Federal agencies could work with the state contact, as the product moves through the state regulatory process, to correct any problems as they arise.

The committee recommends that ONDCP, in cooperation with FDA, DEA, SAMHSA, and NIDA, take an active role in compiling relevant information about state regulatory processes for anti-addiction medications that are categorized as narcotics and educating state regulators and pharmaceutical company representatives about the processes and their practical consequences. To implement that recommendation, the following steps may be taken:

- Conduct a comprehensive study of state laws and regulations pertinent to the development of anti-addiction medications that are controlled substances, and develop a step-by-step manual for pharmaceutical companies explaining the mechanisms involved in launching an anti-addiction medication.
- Establish and maintain on-line access to the comprehensive study, as well as to state regulatory information of a practical nature (for example, a directory of relevant state officials) to facilitate pharmaceutical company access.
- Sponsor nationwide or regional educational meetings for state authorities and clinic administrators to disseminate information about potential anti-addiction medications.

Long-Term Actions

Ultimately, close attention should be given to reforming the current patchwork of state regulations. The committee considered total federal preemption of state controlled-substance laws and regulations insofar as those authorities affect the development of anti-addiction medications, but it concluded that such a proposal would go beyond what is strictly necessary, and could also be politically unrealistic. The committee does believe, however, that the initiative for reform must come from the federal government, and will have to involve some form of legislative change.

The committee recommends, on the basis of the comprehensive study recommended above, that ONDCP, in coordination with other relevant federal agencies, develop a series of specific actions encouraging states to reform their laws and regulations to facilitate the availability of new anti-addiction medications that are controlled substances.[6] Those actions should give particular attention to:

•   Modifying state laws and regulations for narcotic treatment programs to remove the need to reopen and amend the laws or regulations to accommodate each new product.
•   Imposing specific deadlines for state regulatory action in response to FDA approval of a new anti-addiction medication that requires state action to be dispensed to patients.
•   Developing flexible, alternative means of controlling the dispensing of anti-addiction narcotic medications that would avoid the "methadone model" of individually approved treatment centers.

Finally, the committee urges that Congress, in cooperation with the National Conference of Commissioners on Uniform State Laws, draft legislation requiring states to implement needed changes, rather than preempt outright the relevant state laws or regulations. The legislation could establish regulatory benchmarks (such as the length of time allowed after FDA approval for the state to take legislative or other action; types of alternative dispensing controls). That legislation could be freestanding or as an amendment to NATA.

---

[6]ONDCP as previously drafted and put forth model state legislation on numerous topics, thus there is a precedent for model legislation on research and development of anti-addiction medications.

If the federal government wishes to remove regulatory obstacles to the development of anti-addiction medications, then significant changes in current policies, laws, and regulations are necessary (Chapter 8).

MARKET OBSTACLES AND CREATING INCENTIVES

Size of the Market

From the pharmaceutical industry's point of view the size of the potential market for determining investment in research and development (R&D), is not estimated simply from the absolute number of patients with a given condition. For example, there are about 2.1 million cocaine-dependent individuals and 500,000 to 1 million opiate-dependent individuals in the United States (Hunt and Rhodes, 1992; Kreek, 1992). Those numbers are high enough to be attractive, yet there is significantly more pharmaceutical activity in other areas with comparable or much smaller patient populations. Approximately 25,000 individuals have amyotrophic lateral sclerosis (ALS or Lou Gehrig's disease), for which several pharmaceutical companies have compounds in various stages of clinical development (Samotin, 1994). Similarly, the market for medications to treat the 2.1 million epilepsy patients is well established at $400 million to 500 million, and three new products have been or are about to be approved (Samotin, 1994). The pharmaceutical industry appears willing to invest in R&D for markets that are smaller in size or approximately the same size as the cocaine user market, yet reluctant to enter the field of anti-addiction products. There are several reasons for this apparent paradox.

First, there is a perceived lack of a market, by the pharmaceutical industry, in terms of true medical demand, access to patients, and motivation of patients. It is believed that a portion of the population is either not interested in treatment or erratic in compliance. Second, one segment of treatment providers is committed to a "drug-free" concept. Third, any particular medication is likely to be useful for a particular indication (such as reducing the craving for cocaine) and not for treating the entire drug-dependent population. The result is greater uncertainty in predicting the demand or true market size for new anti-addiction medications than for drugs intended for more established markets (Samotin, 1994). However, those niches represent opportunities, especially for small pharmaceutical companies, biotechnology companies, and those already involved in the development of central nervous system (CNS) compounds, that have not been fully explored by the industry. Furthermore, an uncharted market coupled with the limits in the basic science of addiction present a significant obstacle in the discovery and delivery of anti-addiction medications.

The Orphan Drug Act (P.L. 97-414) was enacted to stimulate the market in the development of medications for rare diseases by granting market exclusivity to companies who developed those compounds (Chapter 7). The standard for orphan status is whether a drug is intended to treat a disease or condition that affects fewer than 200,000 persons in the United States or that affects more than 200,000 but for which there is no reasonable expectation of recovering development costs from sales in the United States. Since the passage of the Orphan Drug Act in 1983, the pharmaceutical industry has marketed 60 medications for orphan diseases, and FDA has granted 488 orphan drug designations (Sanders, 1993). The Orphan Drug Act could similarly be used as a mechanism to provide market exclusivity to companies with FDA approved anti-addiction medications. The committee believes that the FDA should consider the actual patient population likely to be treated, rather than that potentially treatable, as there is probably a large segment of the drug-dependent population that will never present for pharmacotherapy. It is illogical and counterproductive to the purposes of the Orphan Drug Act to count those patients against the 200,000 threshold.

The committee recommends that FDA interpret the Orphan Drug Act broadly with the intent of granting orphan drug status to FDA-approved anti-addiction medications whose potential market can reasonably be judged to meet the 200,000 patient criterion stipulated by law. Alternatively, new legislation similar to the Orphan Drug Act could be drafted specifically for FDA-approved anti-addiction medications.

The committee believes that the designation of orphan or orphan like status for approved anti-addiction medications is necessary to stimulate market investment because the financial return is limited, given the nature of the anti-addiction market (Chapter 9).

Drug Pricing and Intellectual Property Rights

In 1986, the Congress passed the Federal Technology and Transfer Act (P.L. 99-502) to encourage private companies to commercialize federal inventions. The statute authorizes federal laboratories to enter into cooperative research and development agreements (CRADAs) with nonprofit institutions and private companies. CRADAs enable government agencies to negotiate exclusive commercialization licenses with industry partners. In 1989, NIH made an administrative decision to adopt a reasonable (or fair) pricing clause[7] into its CRADAS in response to complaints about the introductory price of AZT (zidovudine), an AIDS medication, which was deemed excessive at $10,000 per patient per year. AZT was developed through a cooperative agreement. Such pricing provisions are also included in NIH exclusive licensing agreements.

The potential impact of CRADAs on pricing of products and patent rights has been an important issue of concern for the pharmaceutical industry. Industry representatives have noted that the "reasonable pricing clause" is an important deterrent to a long-term, effective partnership between the government and the private sector. It views the provisions as too broad and too threatening to proprietary interests (U.S. DHHS, 1993).

The committee also heard from industry that the CRADA process is lengthy and complex, often taking about a year for final approval and requiring many layers of review (Chapter 9). Industry officials noted their frustration with the process required to establish a CRADA which, rather than encourage innovative research, acts as another disincentive. NIH is fully aware of the controversy, and is currently reassessing its CRADA policy. There have been two public meetings (July 21 and September 8, 1994) on the issue.

Inasmuch as the language of the "reasonable pricing clause" was adopted by administrative action within NIH and is not legislatively required, NIH could resolve the controversy by administrative action, and, at the same time protect the interests of the public.

The committee recommends that administrative action be taken by NIH to resolve the issue of reasonable pricing in CRADAs. However, if NIH is unsuccessful in stimulating the industry to form cooperative agreements, then the committee recommends legislative action to remove or modify the reasonable pricing clause.

In the absence of a definition of "fair or reasonable price" and in light of NIH's lack of expertise to undertake meaningful analyses of private-sector pricing decisions (OTA, 1993; U.S. DHHS, 1993), the committee believes that this obstacle should be removed. Additionally, NIH should take steps to streamline the CRADA process. NIH could assign additional staff members or establish a centralized committee, to eliminate the need for multiple levels of

---

[7]Section 8.3 of the NIH Patent Policy Board's Model CRADA states, "NIH have a concern that there be a reasonable relationship between the pricing of a licensed product, the public investment in that product, and the health and safety needs of the public. Accordingly, exclusive commercialization licenses granted for NIH intellectual property rights may require that this relationship be supported by reasonable evidence."

review and provide a single site for negotiating and approving CRADAs (IOM Workshop, June 13, 1994).

Societal Stigma

The societal stigma of developing and marketing a medication for the treatment of drug-dependent patients is a concern for pharmaceutical companies. They fear that, once a medication is approved for use in the treatment of drug addiction, the market for other indications will diminish or disappear. Eli Lilly's experience with methadone illustrates the point. Methadone was developed as an analgesic, but its use for pain relief significantly diminished once it became widely used as a treatment for heroin addiction. Patients do not want to take a medication associated with drug addiction. Thus, the pharmaceutical industry is understandably reluctant to develop compounds specifically for drug addiction, if other medical uses for the compound are possible.

There is no easy solution to the problem of stigma associated with drug addiction and its treatment. However, the committee stresses the need for national leadership in support of pharmacotherapy and continued emphasis on prevention and treatment. The sense of stigma is most likely to diminish as a result of public education and broader acceptance of addiction as a treatable disease (Chapter 9).

NEED FOR FEDERAL LEADERSHIP

The committee has considered and attempted to bring clarity to the multiple components involved in the development of anti-addiction medications. Such development depends critically on cooperation between the public and private sectors. Yet the number of federal agencies involved, current agency funding and staffing levels, regulatory requirements, remaining scientific questions, and other issues present difficult challenges to successful partnership and cooperation. Although many of the challenges are addressed in this report, it is important to recognize that government policies have not provided a strong emphasis on pharmacotherapy for the treatment of drug addiction. This lack of federal leadership represents an additional disincentive to industry, in that it affects the public sector's ability to establish clear guidelines, enhance interagency cooperation, and provide research programs with the stability necessary for medication discovery and development (Chapter 9). In addition to its role in developing medications for drug addiction, the government is likely to be the major purchaser of those medications. Thus, government policies are critical in determining the environment in which such medications are developed and are necessary for supporting pharmacotherapy as an important and accepted form of treatment.

The committee applauds the current emphasis on treatment in the 1994 National Drug Control Strategy and suggests an additional action to underscore the importance of treatment and strengthen federal leadership.

One option might be for the President to issue an executive order assigning a high priority to the development of medications for drug-abuse treatment. This, or some other explicit action, would enhance cooperation among the government agencies involved, focus their activities, and aid in the removal of existing institutional barriers.

Explicit action at the Presidential or cabinet level would have the added benefit of signaling to the private sector that the development of anti-addiction medications is a matter of high national priority. The committee further believes that progress in this area should be monitored. Thus, any action taken should include a provision for reporting by the involved agencies regarding their efforts to coordinate with other agencies and remove barriers identified. Examples of specific ways in which cooperation could expedite development of anti-addiction medications are formalization of agreements between NIDA and the Department of Veterans Affairs for support of clinical trials, and encouragement of all agencies to promote cooperation with the private sector. Other strategies, including the use of executive-level task forces and commissions, may also be options to strengthen federal leadership and give the issue high priority in the eyes of both the public and private sectors.

CONCLUSIONS

In reviewing the obstacles presented to the pharmaceutical industry for the development of anti-addiction medications, it is clear that, the disincentives outweigh the incentives. The formidable scientific and marketing issues, regulatory complexities, and financial uncertainties add up to an unattractive picture to the pharmaceutical industry, which tends to enter R&D investment from a high risk-high reward perspective.

Although it is possible to envision incentives that would interest some pharmaceutical companies (e.g., small pharmaceutical companies, biotechnology companies, or those companies already involved in the development of CNS compounds) without strong federal leadership, in establishing the role of pharmacotherapy and a long-term federal commitment to research, the committee believes all other efforts are likely to falter. As the federal government considers policies that will remove obstacles, the committee suggests a tiered approach of incentives, allowing each tier of incentives time to produce the desired effect (Chapter 9). For example, the first action may be the removal of disincentives, then the creation of modest incentives, and finally the development of extraordinary incentives.

The removal of disincentives includes many of the committee's administrative recommendations: use of orphan drug and fast track mechanisms for anti-addiction compounds; removal of adverse effects on clinical research of DEA requirements under the Controlled Substances Act; and counting DEA review time as part of the regulatory process for purposes of patent term extension for controlled substances.

The creation of modest incentives should include broad interpretation of the Orphan Drug Act to include anti-addiction medications or similar legislation to stimulate the market in the development of anti-addiction medications; a strong federal leadership role in support of treatment of drug-dependent patients; funding of basic research and training; adequate funding of treatment; and a modification or elimination of the "reasonable pricing clause" in CRADAs.

Finally, the committee considered two extraordinary incentives that the executive branch and the Congress may wish to consider. They are presented below as options for consideration, and they are not committee recommendations.

OPTIONS FOR FURTHER CONSIDERATION

The committee discussed whether the overall strategy (i.e., strong federal leadership regarding drug abuse treatment and support of research) coupled with removal of obstacles to anti-addiction medication R&D would be likely to result in activity by the pharmaceutical industry. Additionally, the committee considered whether a considerable economic incentive specifically intended to reward the development of new anti-addiction medications was needed. The committee did not reach a consensus on that issue and has no formal recommendation for such an extraordinary incentive.

Nevertheless, the committee wishes to include in this report a brief description of two incentives that were supported by a majority of its members, recognizing that the committee has not provided details for implementation of those incentives (Chapter 9). Both of the following proposals are limited to medications developed for cocaine addiction and are intended to create a guaranteed market in view of the limited potential for return on investment of anti-addiction medications as perceived by the pharmaceutical industry.

Option 1 would offer developers of the first few (e.g., two or three) FDA-approved medications for the treatment of cocaine addiction for 3 years after approval a federal subsidy of a maximum of $50 million for purchase of the drug. The subsidy could be given, for example, through reimbursement of the copayment portion of medications for patients with health insurance and the full cost of medications for those patients without medical insurance.

Option 2 would allow for standing federal purchase orders for prearranged quantities and at an adequate price of one or more new cocaine treatment medications to begin at the time of FDA approval. The purchase orders would establish unambiguous confirmation of a market demand for those products, thereby stimulating investment and commercialization.

The options presented above were favored by a majority of the committee. Most committee members also favored implementation of those extraordinary incentives only if the first two tiers of recommendations fail to stimulate progress in the anti-addiction medications market. A majority of the committee agreed, however, that the above options should be deliberated by the executive branch and Congress as they develop policies to stimulate this area of research and development (Chapter 9).

REFERENCES

Anglin MD, Hser Y. 1992. Treatment of drug abuse. In: Watson RW, ed. Drug Abuse Treatment. New York: Humana Press. Vol. 3, Drug and Alcohol Abuse Reviews.

Gerstein DR, Johnson RA, Harwood HJ, Fountain D, Suter N, Malloy K. 1994. Evaluating Recovery Services: The California Drug and Alcohol Treatment Assessment (CALDATA). Sacramento, CA: California Department of Alcohol and Drug Programs.

Goldstein HM. 1989. The Availability of Methadone Maintenance in California. Drug Abuse Information and Monitoring Project (DAIMP) White Paper Series 9. Los Angeles: UCLA Drug Abuse Research Center, DAIMP. Prepared for the California Department of Alcohol and Drug Programs.

Hunt DE, Rhodes W. 1992. Characteristics of Heavy Cocaine Users Including Polydrug Use, Criminal Activity, and Health Risks. Prepared for the Office of National Drug Control Policy by Abt Associates, Inc.

IOM (Institute of Medicine). 1990. Treating Drug Problems. Gerstein DR, Harwood HJ, eds. Washington, DC: National Academy Press.

IOM (Institute of Medicine). 1995. Federal Regulation of Methadone Treatment. Rettig R, Yarmolinsky A, eds. Washington, DC: National Academy Press.

Kreek MJ. 1992. Rationale for maintenance pharmacotherapy of opiate dependence. In: O'Brien CP, Jaffe JH, eds. Addictive States. New York: Raven Press. 205–230.

NCJA (National Criminal Justice Association). 1991. Guide to State Controlled Substances Acts. Washington, DC: NCJA.

OTA (Office of Technology Assessment). 1990. The Effectiveness of Drug Abuse Treatment: Implications for Controlling AIDS/HIV Infection. Washington, DC: OTA. OTA-BP-H-73. AIDS Related Issues Background Paper 6.

OTA (Office of Technology Assessment). 1993. Pharmaceutical R & D: Costs, Risks and Rewards. Washington, DC: Government Printing Office. OTA-H-522.

Prendergast ML, Anglin MD, Maugh TH, Hser Y. In press. The Effectiveness of Treatment for Drug Abuse. Draft manuscript prepared April 7, 1994 for NIDA Treatment Services Research Branch. Los Angeles: UCLA Drug Abuse Research Center.

Rogowski JA. 1993. Insurance Coverage for Drug Abuse: Private Versus Public Sectors. Santa Monica, CA: RAND. Prepared for the Drug Policy Research Center. MR-166-DPRC.

Samotin S. 1994. Size of the Cocaine Market. Presentation to the IOM Workshop on Policies to Stimulate Private Sector Development of Anti-Addiction Medications. June 13, 1994. Washington, DC. National Academy of Sciences.

Sanders CA. 1993. The Orphan Drug Act: should it be changed? Archives of Internal Medicine 153:2623–2625.

U.S. DHHS (U.S. Department of Health and Human Services), Office of Inspector General. 1993. Technology Transfer and the Public Interest: Cooperative Research and Development Agreements at NIH. OEI-01-92-01100.

1

Introduction

Drug addiction[1] is a highly complex process that involves physiological, behavioral, psychological, and social components. Similarly, its treatment usually takes a multifaceted approach. Methods of treating drug addiction include pharmacotherapy (the use of medications), psychotherapy (group and individual counseling) and social support (such as in the form of employment opportunities and education).

Pharmacotherapy has not received broad support from the federal government, nor has the private sector been active in developing anti-addiction medications. There are many reasons for the apparent lack of support of and activity in this kind of drug development. Clearly, the absence of a large, vocal advocacy group that would voice strong support and lobby for treatment funding and research contributes to the lack of federal leadership and the dearth of anti-addiction medications. But, it should be recognized that drug addiction is a disease (Miller, 1991)—one that is widespread in the United States (there are an estimated 0.5–1 million heroin-dependent individuals and 2.1 million cocaine-dependent individuals) and shows no signs of abating according to national surveys (Hunt and Rhodes, 1992; Kreek, 1992; Johnston et al., 1994a,b)—and like people with any other medical condition, drug addicted individuals deserve to be considered as candidates for medications.

---

[1]Drug addiction is defined as the compulsive use of a drug despite adverse consequences. This report focuses on opiate and cocaine addictions and does not address alcohol and nicotine addictions.

In 1990, the Medications Development Division (MDD) of the National Institute on Drug Abuse (NIDA) was established to support research and development and to work with the private sector to secure Food and Drug Administration (FDA) marketing approval for new medications to treat drug addiction (see mission statement in Appendix B).

This report of the Institute of Medicine (IOM) Committee to Study Medication Development and Research at the National Institute on Drug Abuse focuses on pharmacotherapy for the treatment of drug addiction for several reasons:

- Pharmacotherapy for opiate addiction is successful, and it seems reasonable to assume that effective medications could be useful in treating cocaine addiction.
- Pharmacotherapies will expand the range of treatment options available to physicians and treatment programs (U.S. Congress, Senate, 1989).
- Pharmacotherapies might enhance other treatment modalities.
- Pharmacotherapy might permit more cost-effective outpatient approaches.

Additionally, Congress has specifically required the committee to determine the current conditions for developing anti-addiction medications. The need for pharmacotherapy is further driven by the public-health, economic, and criminal repercussions of illicit drug use (particularly use of opiates and cocaine). The committee focused its attention on medications to treat opiate and cocaine addictions, although it recognizes that the two addictive drugs that are most important with respect to morbidity, mortality, and economic costs are alcohol and nicotine.

This chapter examines the magnitude of the illicit drug-use problem and its effects on society. Chapter 2 examines the state of scientific knowledge concerning the mechanisms of drug addiction and the difficulty of developing anti-addiction medications. The work of NIDA's MDD is discussed in Chapter 3. Chapters 4–9 focus on the disincentives faced by the pharmaceutical industry in developing anti-addiction medications—treatment financing, physician training and education, federal and state regulation, and market issues—and present policy and legislative solutions.

PUBLIC-HEALTH REPERCUSSIONS OF ILLICIT DRUG USE

Drug addiction has both individual and societal ramifications. Overall societal trends in drug-addiction policy have ranged from minimal libertarian approaches in the middle 1800s to medical and criminal approaches that have alternated in emphasis since the late 1800s (IOM, 1990). Current government approaches are both medical and criminal, involving federal expenditures for drug enforcement and interdiction and federal, state, and private expenditures for drug treatment and drug-addiction research (IOM, 1990).

Historical analysis has demonstrated that policy trends are driven by various factors, including the social class of drug-users, prevailing perceptions regarding the causes of drug addiction (e.g., personal choice, physiological dependence, moral weakness, and genetic predisposition), the limited availability of effective treatments (e.g., methadone), and the relation of the costs of drug-related violence to the public-health costs of drug addiction. Increasingly violence itself is being viewed as a public-health problem as evidenced by increasing public support of antiviolence initiatives in the agencies of the Department of Health and Human Services (DHHS), such as the Centers for Disease Control and Prevention (CDC). This shift coincides with a well-defined relationship between drug addiction and the acquired immune deficiency syndrome (AIDS) epidemic; mounting data on the role of drug addiction in the alarming rise of tuberculosis (TB), particularly the often intractable and deadly drug-resistant form; and the increase in the number of drug-exposed infants. Thus, the development of anti-addiction medications to treat illicit drug use has ramifications not only for addicted individuals, but also for society at large.

Health Consequences: Violence

Violence is now accepted as one of the major public-health problems facing the United States[2], and the CDC has given the prevention of violence one of its highest priorities (Koop and Lundberg, 1992; Rosenberg et al., 1992; Schneider et al., 1992). Violence and illicit drug use are inextricably linked through several scenarios: the "turf battles" of drug sale and drug distribution, the criminal and often violent behavior prompted by the need for money to support drug use, and the violence (often domestic) associated with the pharmacological effects of some drugs on the drug-addicted individual (BJS, 1992; Marwick, 1992). In the illegal drug business, violence is systemic and is the typical interaction used to protect and expand markets and deal with competitors, with buyers or sellers suspected of cheating, and with police or witnesses (BJS, 1992).

---

[2]Violence has many causes, including the direct behavioral disinhibiting effects of alcohol. Of state prison inmates surveyed who were convicted of committing homicide, 25 percent reported being under the influence of alcohol at the time of the offense (BJS, 1993).

In the circular nature of the drug-crime relationship, persons with criminal records are more likely than persons without criminal records to report being drug-users, and drug-users report greater involvement with crime (BJS, 1992). In a 1991 survey of state-prison inmates, 28 percent of inmates incarcerated for violent crimes reported committing the crimes while under the influence of drugs, and 27 percent reported committing robbery to obtain money to buy drugs (BJS, 1993). Data from the 1991 Drug Use Forecasting Program (a 24-city program involving interviews and urine-tests of a sample of arrested persons) indicate that 65 percent of males arrested for robbery and 48 percent of males arrested for homicide had evidence of illicit drug use in their urine (NIJ, 1992). Data on arrested females show even higher percentages—76 percent arrested for robbery, 50 percent arrested for assault, and 65 percent arrested for homicide had evidence of illicit drug use in their urine (NIJ, 1992). Cocaine was the most prevalent drug, with percentages as high as 62 percent of arrested males in Manhattan and Philadelphia (NIJ, 1992). Violence and drug use are also connected through drugs' pharmacological activity—especially that of such stimulants as cocaine, crack cocaine, phencyclidine (PCP), and amphetamines—which can produce irritability, paranoia, and a "need for action" that increases the likelihood of violence (Miller et al., 1991; BJS, 1992; Marwick, 1992). The links between violence and drug addiction add to the seriousness of the public-health need for effective treatment of drug addiction.

Health Consequences: AIDS

Injection of illicit drugs is the second most common risk behavior associated with the spread of AIDS, and in some sections of the U.S. recent data show that heterosexual drug users account for the largest group of new AIDS cases (CDC, 1994; Goldstein, 1994). More than one-third (37 percent) of AIDS cases reported from June 1993 through June 1994 were related to injection of illicit drugs through the sharing of contaminated injection equipment, through heterosexual contact with an injecting drug-user (IDU), or through maternal injection of drugs (Table 1.1) (CDC, 1994). In women, the percentages of AIDS cases involving injection of illicit drugs are alarmingly high. Of the 51,235 female AIDS cases reported to CDC through June 1994 almost half (24,660 cases) were attributable to injection of illicit drugs and another 19 percent (9,976 cases) to sex with infected IDU partners (CDC, 1994). The current prevalence of the human immunodeficiency virus (HIV) in the estimated 1.1–1.8 million IDUs is unknown (OTA, 1990). However, of those in treatment programs, an estimated 61,000–398,000 IDUs are infected with HIV; the estimates vary in different regions of the United States and reach a high of 65 percent in New York City (OTA, 1990; Hahn et al., 1989).

TABLE 1.1 AIDS Cases Related to Injection of Illicit Drugs (Percentage of total cases)

Exposure Category	Cases Reported June 1993–June 1994		Cumulative Total Reported	
Injecting drug use:				
Men	17,441	(20.5)	73,705	(18.3)
Women	6,138	(7)	24,660	(6)
Heterosexual contact with an injecting drug user:				
Men	959	(1)	4,263	(1)
Women	2,197	(3)	9,976	(2.5)
Men who have sex with men and inject drugs	4,165	(5)	25,447	(6)
Pediatric cases (<13 years old): Mother who is an injecting drug user	284	(0.3)	2,192	(0.5)
Mother who has sex with an injecting drug user	137	(0.2)	969	(0.2)
Total cases related to injecting drug use	31,321	(37)	141,212	(35)
Total cases reported	85,260		401,749	

SOURCE: CDC, 1994.

AIDS and illicit drug use are linked not only by injection drug use, but also through an increase in high-risk sexual behaviors and perinatal transmission of HIV. Such behaviors include exchange of sex for drugs, unprotected sex and multiple partners, and prostitution to gain money to buy drugs (Turner et al., 1989). Heroin and cocaine alone or in combination are the most common injectable drugs, although some injection of amphetamines has also been reported (OTA, 1990). Of the 5,734 cases of AIDS in children under 13 years old reported to CDC through June 1994, 89 percent are attributable to perinatal HIV transmission (CDC, 1994). Most (55 percent) of the pediatric AIDS cases are associated with injection of illicit drugs—38 percent with maternal injection of drugs and 17 percent with maternal sexual contact with an IDU (CDC, 1994). All infants born to HIV-infected mothers carry passively acquired maternal antibodies that make them HIV-seropositive, and an estimated 25–35 percent of these infants are actually infected (Hardy, 1991).

Health Consequences: Tuberculosis

TB was once a major public-health problem in the United States that caused many deaths, but it declined with the discovery of effective medications and with increased public-health screening and intervention programs. TB is an infectious bacterial disease that commonly affects the lungs (pulmonary type) but can also affect other organ systems (systemic type). It is again an immediate threat to the well-being of thousands of Americans who are homeless, live in poverty, take illicit drugs, or are infected with HIV. The very factors that are contributing most greatly to the increase in TB also present severe challenges to stemming its further spread (OTA, 1993). For example, CDC recently reported that nearly 23 percent of inmates in correctional facilities had positive skin tests for TB (CDC, 1993a). The closed nature of the prison environment, coupled with overcrowding, makes prisons ideal for transmission of TB. Prisons also have a high concentration of people from environments of poverty, and the inmate population has a high prevalence of drug addiction. Most inmates will re-enter the community, and failures of the prison health system will have impacts outside the prison walls.

The emergence of TB strains that are resistant to many of the standard medications exacerbates the threat. From 1985 to 1992, rates of TB increased significantly in people 25–44 years old (54.5 percent increase), Hispanics (74.5 percent increase), and African-Americans (26.8 percent increase) (CDC, 1993b). TB has also increased greatly in children, presumably in part through transmission from older family members (CDC, 1993b). Drug-resistant TB is high among IDUs and those infected with HIV. Positive skin tests for TB have been found in nearly 10 percent of patients in drug-treatment programs (CDC, 1993a). The incidence of TB among those with HIV is almost 500 times that in the non-HIV-infected population (Barnes et al., 1991). That is an ominous figure because people in the later, more severe stages of AIDS often do not test positive for TB in standard skin tests, even if they have active TB (Barnes et al., 1991; Braun et al., 1993); thus, simple screening procedures are often inaccurate, and this increases the threat of TB transmission to health-care workers.

It is clear from a public-health perspective that illicit drug use and its associated risks of HIV and TB are serious threats to the health of non-drug-addicted populations that justify the investment of federal funds in drug-treatment research and prevention. The burden of HIV and TB on the health-care system is important to consider. For example, the CDC spent about $20 million per year for TB programs in 1967, 1968, and 1969. The expenditure fell dramatically in 1972–1983 but increased to $100 million in 1993, mainly because of HIV-related programs (OTA, 1993). The average cost of medication to treat uncomplicated TB is about $350 per person, but medications for a case of drug resistant TB cost an average of $8,720 and possibly as much as $35,000 (OTA, 1993).

Health Consequences: Drug-exposed Infants

NIDA's recently released National Pregnancy and Health Survey provides nationally representative data on the extent of drug use during pregnancy (NIDA, 1994). The survey estimated that 221,000 women (with 220,000 live births) used one or more illicit drugs during pregnancy with estimates of 45,100 women having used cocaine (34,800 of those women used crack cocaine) and 3,600 women having used heroin during pregnancy.

Drug-exposed infants have more medical complications and longer hospital stays after birth and possibly suffer from long-term developmental deficits (GAO, 1990). Fetal effects of maternal illicit drug use are difficult to separate, however, from the many risk factors often present in the lives of drug-using women, such as infrequent or no prenatal care, poor nutrition, low socioeconomic status, low maternal age, and multiple drug use, including cigarette-smoking and alcohol. Frequency of drug use, timing of drug use during pregnancy, drug purity, and dosage are additional confounding variables.

Cocaine acts as a vasoconstrictor (possibly constricting blood vessels in the placenta and umbilical cord), and its maternal use during pregnancy has been found to be associated with impaired fetal growth and lower head size at birth (Finnegan and Kandall, 1992). Studies are ongoing to determine the relationship between prenatal cocaine exposure and birth defects, preterm birth, and neonatal neurobehavioral dysfunction, including heightened sensitivity and irritability, abnormal sleep patterns, and decreased interactive behavior (Peters and Theorell, 1990; Zuckerman, 1991). Maternal use of opiates increases the likelihood of low birth weight, prematurity, small fetal head size, and sudden infant death syndrome (Zuckerman, 1991; Finnegan and Kandall, 1992). Infants of opiate-addicted mothers often are addicted and go through the neonatal abstinence syndrome in withdrawal (Kronstadt, 1991). Long-term developmental consequences of in utero exposure to illicit drugs—including language, behavioral, and learning difficulties—are being studied (Kronstadt, 1991; Zuckerman, 1991).

ECONOMIC COSTS OF ILLICIT DRUG USE TO SOCIETY

Given the extent of the major health consequences associated with illicit drug use, the need for treatment, including effective pharmacotherapy, is urgent. In addition to the public-health imperative for developing these medications, the economic costs associated with use of illicit drugs are staggering.

It has been estimated that about $66.9 billion (Table 1.2) was spent in 1990 in dealing with some aspect of illicit drug use (D. Rice, University of California at San Francisco, personal communication). That figure includes costs for health are, for drug-addiction treatment and prevention, for fighting and preventing drug-related crime, and for resources lost because of reduced worker productivity or death (Figure 1.1). These costs have steadily and substantially risen from an estimated $44 billion in 1985 to $58 billion in 1988 and to the 1990 estimates in excess of $66 billion (Rice et al., 1991; Rice, UCSF, personal communication). Although the focus of this report is on heroin and cocaine, economic costs are not available for specific drugs, so the data cited here include all illicit drug use.

TABLE 1.2 Estimated Economic Costs of Drug Abuse, 1990

Type of Cost	Amount ($ millions)	Percent Distribution
Total	**66,873**	**100.0**
Core Costs	**14,602**	**21.8**
Direct	3,197	4.8
Mental health organizations	867	1.3
Short stay hospitals	1,889	2.8
Office-based physicians	88	0.1
Other professional services	32	0.05
Support costs	321	0.5
Indirect	11,405	17.1
Morbidity[a]	7,997	12.0
Mortality	3,408	5.1
Other related costs	**45,989**	**68.8**
Direct	18,043	27.0
Crime	18,035	27.0
Social-welfare administration	8	0.01
Indirect	27,946	41.8
Victims of crime	1,042	1.6
Incarceration	7,813	11.7
Crime careers	19,091	28.5
AIDS	**6,282**	**9.4**

NOTE: Within each category are direct costs, for which payment is made, and indirect costs, for which resources are lost. 1990 costs based on socioeconomic indexes applied to 1985 estimates.

[a]Defined by the author as the value of goods and services lost by individuals unable to perform their usual activities because of drug abuse, or unable to perform them at a level of full effectiveness (Rice et al., 1990). SOURCE: D. Rice, University of California at San Francisco, personal communication.

Drug-related crime cost society over $46 billion in 1990 and constitutes the highest percentage of the economic burden placed on society as a result of illicit drug use (Table 1.2). This figure is a composite of the direct costs of police protection, drug-traffic control, property destruction, and legal adjudication and the indirect costs of lost productivity for victims of crime and for those incarcerated in prisons or involved in criminal careers. Direct health-related costs of illicit drug use were estimated to have totaled over $3 billion in 1990, and health-care costs due to the large number of AIDS cases associated with injection drug use were estimated at $6.3 billion in 1990 (Table 1.2). Other costs of illicit drug use include morbidity costs (the value of reduced or lost productivity due to drug use) and mortality costs (the value of productivity lost because of premature death resulting from drug addiction); these indirect costs were estimated to total over $11 billion in 1990 in the United States. The social-welfare costs summarized in Table 1.2 (estimated at $8 million in 1990) include costs of public assistance, food stamps, unemployment insurance, and other social-welfare programs.

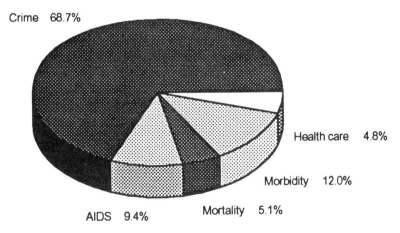

FIGURE 1.1 Summary of the economic cost of illicit drug use, 1990. Percentage breakdown of $66.9 billion cost of U.S. illicit drug use in 1990. SOURCE: D. Rice, University of California at San Francisco, personal communication.

Those estimates include federal expenditures. In 1992, the federal government spent $11.9 billion on drug control and employed 66,652 persons (full-time equivalents) to work in various agencies on the illicit drug-use problem (ONDCP, 1992). The Department of Justice handled 36 percent of the 1992 expenditure, DHHS received 17 percent, and the Department of Defense received

11 percent (ONDCP, 1992). Total drug-control expenditures by the federal government have increased by more than 750 percent from 1981 to 1993 (ONDCP, 1992).

U.S. national drug-control policy has focused primarily on supply reduction; about two-thirds of drug-control expenditure has gone for interdiction, intelligence, incarceration, and other law-enforcement activities (ONDCP, 1992). The remaining one-third of the federal drug-control expenditure has been divided among research and development, treatment, and prevention (Figure 1.2). The percentage for research and development has remained virtually unchanged since 1981, varying from 3.5 to 5 percent of the total expenditure (ONDCP, 1992). While there have been increases in the amount spent on treatment and prevention, the percentage of the total drug-control budget spent for treatment has been halved from 30 percent in 1981 to a low of 16 percent in 1992.

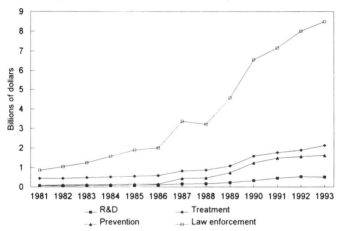

FIGURE 1.2 Federal drug control budget trends (1981–1993). NOTE: Figures are in current dollars. SOURCE: ONDCP, 1992.

The 1994 national drug-control strategy proposed substantial increases in spending for treatment, and reductions in the percentage spent on law-enforcement supply control efforts (Washington Post, 1994). The strategy called for increasing the availability of treatment by providing $355 million in new block grants to states, with the target of treating an additional 140,000 heavy drug users each year. However, the final legislation approved only a $57 million increase for state block grants in the FY95 budget.

EXTENT OF ILLICIT DRUG USE

The widespread presence of illicit drug use in the United States is document-ed in surveys of households, students, and jail and prison inmates (Table 1.3). National incidence of illicit drug use was highest in the 1970s (although cocaine use peaked in the 1980s) and has steadily declined in the past 20 years. However, a recent survey of junior-high-school and high-school students shows indications that this decline has halted and there may be a small upturn in illicit drug use (Johnston et al., 1994a). Of 1993 high-school seniors surveyed, 42.9 percent reported ever using illicit drugs, and 18.3 percent reported use in the preceding month, predominantly marijuana use (Johnston et al., 1994a). Similarly, 14.9 percent of young adults reported using any illicit drug in the preceding month (Johnston et al., 1994b). Household, prison and jail, and school surveys result in the following data:[3]

- An estimated 77 million Americans have used an illicit drug at some time in their life (SAMHSA, 1994c).
- An estimated 24.4 million Americans have used an illicit drug within the last year (SAMHSA, 1994c).
- An estimated 11.7 million Americans have used an illicit drug within the last month (SAMHSA, 1994c). Of 1993 high-school seniors surveyed, 18.3 percent reported use of an illicit drug in the last month—a substantial increase from the 14.4 percent of 1992 high-school seniors (Johnston et al., 1994a).
- Marijuana, the most commonly used illicit drug in the United States, has been tried by nearly one-third of all Americans, with highest preceding year use in those 18–25 years old (22.9 percent had used marijuana in 1993). Of the 18.6 million Americans estimated to have used marijuana in 1993, 5.1 million are estimated to have used it weekly (SAMHSA, 1994c).
- An estimated 4.5 million Americans used cocaine in 1993 (SAMH-SA, 1994c). The number of heavy cocaine users, using at least once a week, is estimated at 2.1 million (Hunt and Rhodes, 1992). Crack, a smokable form of cocaine, is estimated to have been used by 996,000 Americans in the last year (SAMHSA, 1994c).
- Heroin statistics are more difficult to obtain from nationwide surveys because heroin use involves less than 1 percent of the population

---

[3]Note that a recent General Accounting Office report warns that use figures, particularly in household and student surveys, are underestimated in that these surveys have high nonresponse rates and do not include high-risk groups, such as high-school dropouts (GAO, 1993).

and many heroin-users are not part of a traditional household environment. It is estimated that there are 1 million recent or frequent heroin-users, including 0.5 million heroin-addicted individuals (Kreek, 1992).

Drug use was a direct or contributing factor in 7,532 deaths reported in 1992 to the Drug Abuse Warning Network (DAWN) by 137 medical examiner facilities in 38 metropolitan areas. Cocaine was the most frequently reported drug (46 percent), alcohol in combination with other drugs was mentioned in 39 percent of the cases, and heroin or morphine in 39 percent (SAMHSA, 1994b). Morbidity reports from DAWN indicate that there were about 433,493 drug abuse-related hospital emergency-room episodes in 1992 (SAMHSA, 1994a). Alcohol in combination with other drugs was mentioned most frequently, in nearly one-third of all episodes (more than one drug per episode can be mentioned), followed in frequency by cocaine (28 percent), and heroin or morphine (11 percent). Data collection difficulties including changes in sample composition, nonresponse from data collectors, changes in data collectors, and coding errors, place limitations on interpreting the DAWN data.

ROLE OF PHARMACOTHERAPY

Given the magnitude of the illicit-drug-use problem, and its economic and public-health consequences, addressing this issue requires a dedicated effort not only to develop pharmacotherapies but also to foster prevention, education, and the use of other kinds of treatment. Pharmacotherapy, as an adjunct to other treatment modalities, has not received widespread support, in part because of the lack of patient advocacy and the belief espoused by some that to treat drug addiction with a medication is merely to substitute one drug for another. That belief stems largely from the use of methadone maintenance for opiate-addicted individuals and, although it's a common view, should not be allowed to detract from the proven success of methadone maintenance programs, which have allowed many people to become functional and productive (IOM, 1990; OTA, 1990), or to dominate thinking about the treatment of all types of addictions. Drug addiction is a disease that merits medication for its treatment, like such other chronic diseases as hypertension, diabetes, and cancer (Miller, 1991). That such treatment might not treat root causes of the illness or offer a permanent cure does not detract from the value of pharmacotherapy in improving both quality of life and mortality in patients with those diseases.

TABLE 1.3 Percentages of Drug Users Based on Surveys of Various Populations

Surveys	Any Illicit Drug Use		Cocaine Use		Heroin Use	
	Ever Used	Used in the Preceding Month	Ever Used	Used in the Preceding Month	Ever Used	Used in the Preceding Month
National Household Survey on Drug Abuse (1993)[a]						
Total Population	37.2	5.6	11.3	0.6	1.1	NA
12–17 years old	17.9	6.6	1.1	0.4	0.2	NA
18–25 years old	50.9	13.5	12.5	1.5	0.7	NA
26–34 years old	61.1	8.5	25.6	1.0	1.6	NA
35+ years old	29.9	2.8	8.5	0.4	1.2	NA
Monitoring the Future Study						
12th-grad students[b]	42.9	18.3	6.1	1.3	1.1	0.2
College students[c]	45.9	15.1	6.3	0.7	0.6	<0.05
Young adults[c]	59.6	14.9	16.9	1.4	0.9	0.1
Worldwide Survey of Substance Abuse and Health Behaviors Among Military Personal[d]						
Active-duty military personnel	NA	3.4	NA	0.7	NA	0[d]
Survey of Jail Inmates[e]						
Inmates in 424 local jails	78	44	50	24	18	7
Survey in State Prison Inmates[f]						
Inmates in 277 prison facilities	79	50	50	25	25	10

SOURCE: [a] SAMHSA, 1994c; [b] Johnston et al., 1994a; [c] Johnston et al., 1994b; [d] Bray et al., 1992, estimates round to zero; [e] BJS, 1991, data on "ever used" are for all jail inmates surveyed; data on preceding month use (month before the offense was committed) are for convicted jail inmates; [f] BJS, 1993, data on preceding month use is for the month before the offense was committed. NA=data not available.

Many illnesses combine both biological and behavioral components. Cardiovascular disease, for example, can be caused by an inherited tendency toward high cholesterol concentrations and be exacerbated by eating habits that increase dietary fat intake. Its treatment often consists of interventions to change the diet and, when necessary, drugs to lower cholesterol concentration. Similarly, the optimal treatment in diabetes might involve a combination of dietary management and drug therapy; some people do well with dietary management alone, others need a combination of dietary management and oral antidiabetes drugs or insulin. Likewise, some opiate-addicted individuals do well with supportive therapy after only a short time on methadone; others require methadone therapy for the rest of their life.

Whether the methadone model will apply directly to other addictive drugs, such as cocaine, is not clear. Cocaine is a more complex drug pharmacologically, and a good substitute that is less abusable has not yet been found. The important point is that there is no inherent reason why pharmacological therapy cannot play as important a role in the treatment of drug addiction as other medicinal agents do in the treatment of heart disease, diabetes, and a host of other illnesses.

The pharmaceutical industry has not responded to this urgent need. Since the 1960s and the acceptance of methadone as the treatment of choice for opiate addiction, no pharmacotherapies for cocaine addiction have been approved, and only in the last 10 years have two medications been approved for opiate addiction (levo-alpha-acetylmethadol [LAAM] and naltrexone).

In an effort to determine the status of pharmaceutical industry participation in the development of anti-addiction medications, the committee queried the FDA about the numbers of companies submitting investigational new drug applications (INDs) for anti-addiction medications. FDA's response indicates that there are six pharmaceutical companies with INDs for medications to treat opiate or cocaine addiction (C. Moody, FDA, personal communication). Currently there are 37 INDs for the treatment of drug addiction, but only 18 different drugs are represented. The FDA reports that 5 or 6 INDs are entering phase III clinical trials, however only one IND represents a new substance. Three companies have submitted new drug applications (NDAs) for anti-addiction medications.

The committee was asked to determine the reasons for the lack of activity in the development of anti-addiction medications. It became evident that many factors contribute, including: an inadequate science base on addiction and the prevention of relapse (especially for cocaine); an uncertain market environment (which includes such issues as: treatment financing, lack of trained specialists for the treatment of drug addiction, federal and state regulations, market size, pricing issues, societal stigma, liability issues, difficulties in conducting clinical research); and a lack of sustained federal leadership. Although for a certain segment of the pharmaceutical industry (e.g., small companies, biotechnology companies, or those companies already involved in the development of central nervous system medications) there may be an interest with suitable incentives to proceed with development of anti-addiction medications.

Chapter 2 examines the state of the scientific knowledge concerning opiate and cocaine addiction, the approaches used by NIDA's Medications Development Division to discover medications for cocaine addiction, and the advantages and limitations of those approaches. In Chapter 3, the background and progress of MDD are addressed. Chapters 4-9 examine the obstacles and disincentives faced by the private sector in the development of anti-addiction medications and policy and legislative solutions are presented. Chapters 4 and 5 address drug-abuse treatment—the setting, effectiveness, cost-effectiveness, and the impact of treatment financing on drug development. The need for increased training and education of both specialists and primary care physicians in drug-abuse research and treatment is the focus of Chapter 6. The following two chapters examine the extent and impact of federal (Chapter 7) and state (Chapter 8) laws and regulations on anti-addiction medication development, marketing, and treatment. The report concludes in Chapter 9 with a discussion of additional marketing obstacles, leadership issues, and outlines steps necessary for increasing private sector involvement in the development of anti-addiction medications.

REFERENCES

Barnes PF, Bloch AB, Davidson PT, Snider DE Jr. 1991. Tuberculosis in patients with human immunodeficiency virus infection. New England Journal of Medicine 324:1644–1650.
BJS (Bureau of Justice Statistics). 1991. Drugs and Jail Inmates, 1989. Washington, DC: BJS.
BJS (Bureau of Justice Statistics). 1992. Drugs, Crime, and the Justice System. Washington, DC: Government Printing Office. NCJ-1335652.
BJS (Bureau of Justice Statistics). 1993. Survey of State Prison Inmates, 1991. Washington, DC: BJS. NCJ-136949.
Braun MM, Cote TR, Rabkin CS. 1993. Trends in death with tuberculosis during the AIDS era. Journal of the American Medical Association 269:2865–2868.
Bray RM, Kroutil LA, Luckey JW, Wheeless SC, Iannacchione VG, Anderson DW, Marsden ME, Dunteman GH. 1992. 1992 Worldwide Survey of Substance Abuse and Health Behaviors Among Military Personnel. Research Triangle Park, NC: Research Triangle Institute. RTI/5154/06-16FR.
CDC (Centers for Disease Control and Prevention). 1993a. Tuberculosis prevention in drug-treatment centers and correctional facilities: selected U.S. cities, 1990–1991. Morbidity and Mortality Weekly Report 42:210–213.
CDC (Centers for Disease Control and Prevention). 1993b. Tuberculosis morbidity: United States, 1992. Morbidity and Mortality Weekly Report 42:696–704.
CDC (Centers for Disease Control and Prevention). 1994. HIV/AIDS Surveillance Report 6(1):8–12.

Finnegan LP, Kandall SR. 1992. Maternal and neonatal effects of alcohol and drugs. In: Lowinson JH, Ruiz P, Millman RB, eds. Substance Abuse: A Comprehensive Textbook. 2nd ed. Baltimore: Williams & Wilkins.

GAO (General Accounting Office). 1990. Drug-Exposed Infants: A Generation at Risk. Washington, DC: GAO. GAO HRD-90-138.

GAO (General Accounting Office). 1993. Drug Use Measurement, Strengths, Limitations, and Recommendations for Improvement. Washington, DC: GAO. GAO PEMD-93-18.

Goldstein A. 1994. Most new cases of AIDS in D.C. hit drug users. Washington Post, December 1, 1994:A1.

Hahn RA, Onorato IM, Jones TS, Dougherty J. 1989. Prevalence of HIV infection among intravenous drug users in the United States. Journal of the American Medical Association 261:2677–2684.

Hardy LM. 1991. HIV Screening of Pregnant Women and Newborns. Washington, DC: National Academy Press.

Hunt DE, Rhodes W. 1992. Characteristics of Heavy Cocaine Users Including Polydrug Use, Criminal Activity, and Health Risks. Prepared for the Office of National Drug Control Policy by Abt Associates, Inc.

IOM (Institute of Medicine). 1990. Treating Drug Problems. Gerstein DR, Harwood HJ, eds. Washington, DC: National Academy Press.

Johnston LD, O'Malley PM, Bachman JG. 1994a. National Survey Results on Drug Use from The Monitoring the Future Study, 1975–1993. Vol. I, Secondary School Students. Rockville, MD: NIDA. NIH Publication No. 94-3809.

Johnston LD, O'Malley PM, Bachman JG. 1994b. National Survey Results on Drug Use from The Monitoring the Future Study, 1975–1993. Vol. II, College Students and Young Adults. Rockville, MD: NIDA. NIH Publication No. 94-3810.

Koop CE, Lundberg GD. 1992. Violence in America: a public health emergency. Journal of the American Medical Association 267:3075–3076.

Kreek MJ. 1992. Rationale for maintenance pharmacotherapy of opiate dependence. In: O'Brien CP, Jaffe JH, eds. Addictive States. New York: Raven Press. 205–230.

Kronstadt D. 1991. Complex developmental issues of prenatal drug exposure. The Future of Children 1:35–49.

Marwick C. 1992. Guns, drugs threaten to raise public health problem of violence to epidemic. Journal of the American Medical Association 267:2993.

Miller NS. 1991. Drug and alcohol addiction as a disease. In: Miller NS, ed. Comprehensive Handbook of Drug and Alcohol Addiction. New York: Marcel Dekker. 295–310.

Miller NS, Gold MS, Mahler JC. 1991. Violent behaviors associated with cocaine use: possible pharmacological mechanisms. International Journal of Addiction 26:1077–1088.

NIDA (National Institute on Drug Abuse). 1994. National Pregnancy and Health Survey. Prepared by Westat, Inc. Rockville, MD: NIDA.

NIJ (National Institute of Justice). 1992. Drug Use Forecasting 1991 Annual Report. Washington, DC: NIJ. NCJ 137776.

ONDCP (Office of National Drug Control Policy). 1992. National Drug Control Strategy: A Nation Responds to Drug Use. Budget Summary. Washington, DC: ONDCP.

OTA (Office of Technology Assessment). 1990. The Effectiveness of Drug Abuse Treatment: Implications for Controlling AIDS/HIV Infection. Washington, DC: OTA. OTA-BP-H-73. AIDS Related Issues Background Paper 6.

OTA (Office of Technology Assessment). 1993. The Continuing Challenge of Tuberculosis. Washington, DC: U.S. Government Printing Office. OTA-H-574.

Peters H, Theorell CJ. 1990. Fetal and neonatal effects of maternal cocaine use. Journal of Obstetric, Gynecologic, and Neonatal Nursing 20: 121–126.

Rice DP, Kelman S, Miller LS, Dunmeyer S. 1990. The Economic Costs of Alcohol and Drug Abuse and Mental Illness: 1985. San Francisco: University of California, Institute for Health and Aging. DHHS Publication No. (ADM) 90-1694.

Rice DP, Kelman S, Miller LS. 1991. Estimates of economic costs of alcohol and drug abuse and mental illness, 1985 and 1988. Public Health Reports 106:280–292.

Rosenberg ML, O'Carroll PW, Powell KE. 1992. Let's be clear violence is a public health problem. Journal of the American Medical Association 267:3071–3072.

SAMHSA (Substance Abuse and Mental Health Services Administration). 1994a. Annual Emergency Room Data 1992. Data from the Drug Abuse Warning Network Series 1, Number 12-A. Rockville, MD: NIDA. DHHS Publication No. (SMA) 94-2080.

SAMHSA (Substance Abuse and Mental Health Services Administration). 1994b. Annual Medical Examiner Data 1992. Data from the Drug Abuse Warning Network Series 1, Number 12-B. Rockville, MD: NIDA. DHHS Publication No. (SMA) 94-2081.

SAMHSA (Substance Abuse and Mental Health Services Administration, Office of Applied Statistics). 1994c. Preliminary Estimates From the 1993 National Household Survey on Drug Abuse. Rockville, MD: SAMHSA. Advance Report Number 7, July 1994.

Schneider D, Greenberg MR, Choi D. 1992. Violence as a public health priority for black Americans. Journal of the National Medical Association 84:843–848.

Turner CF, Miller HG, Moses LE. 1989. AIDS, Sexual Behavior and Intravenous Drug Use. Washington, DC: National Academy Press.

U.S. Congress, Senate. 1989. Committee on the Judiciary. Staff Report. Pharmacotherapy: A Strategy for the 1990's. 101st Cong., 1st sess. S. Prt. 101-000.

U.S. DHHS (U.S. Department of Health and Human Services). 1992. Maternal Drug Abuse and Drug Exposed Children: A Compendium of HHS Activities. Washington, DC: GPO. DHHS Publication No. (ADM) 92-1948.

Washington Post. 1994. Clinton drug policy focuses on treating hard-core users. Washington Post. February 9, 1994. A6.

Zuckerman B. 1991. Drug-exposed infants: understanding the medical risk. The Future of Children 1:28–35.

2

Overview of the State of Scientific Knowledge Concerning Drug Addiction

This chapter focuses on opiates and cocaine, the two classes of drugs targeted by the National Institute on Drug Abuse (NIDA) Medications Development Division (MDD), and begins with an overview of the various concepts of addiction that influence not only the current addiction-treatment methods, but also the scientific investigation of current and potential pharmacological approaches to treatment. For each of the two drug classes, an overview of current scientific knowledge is presented. The remainder of the chapter discusses the MDD cocaine-medication screening program and other strategies for the discovery of an anti-cocaine medication. Conclusions and recommendations are presented with reference to the specific activities of MDD.

CONCEPTS OF DRUG ADDICTION

The initiating event leading to drug addiction is the administration of an agent, such as heroin or cocaine, to obtain a pleasurable effect. Repeated administration can result in addiction defined by compulsive drug-seeking behavior, loss of control over drug use, return to drug use despite repeated efforts to stop, interference with social functioning, and often, impairments to health. Addiction can be associated with the presence of tolerance or sensitization to the effects of the drug and/or dependence, as evidenced by withdrawal symptoms if the drug is abruptly stopped. The two most important psychiatric diagnostic classification schemes, *Diagnostic and Statistical Manual* (APA, 1987) and *International Classification of Diseases* (ICD-10 draft; WHO, 1990), emphasize compulsive drug-seeking and drug-taking behavior, rather than tolerance, dependence, and withdrawal (see Appendix C for diagnostic criteria). However, pharmacological definitions used in the scientific literature require the latter symptoms to be present, and most opiate-addicted patients (although not cocaine-addicted patients) seeking treatment, in fact, exhibit these symptoms.

Drug addiction involves a complex interplay of psychological, physiological, and social mechanisms, and various models have been put forward to account for these mechanisms (Jaffe, 1992). Figure 2.1 presents the schematic model of drug dependence developed by the World Health Organization (WHO), which emphasizes individual and social antecedents and consequences. Such a model is extremely useful, in that it offers numerous points at which interventions can be made to prevent the establishment or break the cycle of drug dependence through both individual and social means. Jaffe (1992) found it useful to modify this scheme in two ways to emphasize more clearly aspects that might affect the urge to engage in use of addictive drugs and aspects that might underlie successful treatment or cessation of drug addiction (Figures 2.2 and 2.3).

Although development of effective anti-addiction medications is only one component of the multifaceted approach needed to develop an effective national strategy for drug-addiction treatment, this report focuses on the development of pharmacological interventions, so the models emphasizing biological factors are presented here. An established working model to account for drug addiction is the "brain-reward hypothesis"—i.e., a neural network is responsible for the subjective experience of pleasure (Koob, 1992; Wise and Hoffman, 1992), and drugs are abused after initial exposure because they activate the brain's reward system. The neurons in the brain, particularly those in the regions comprising the mesolimbic dopamine system (so called because it uses the neurotransmitter dopamine) are thought to be prominent in the rewarding actions of drugs (Koob, 1992). It is likely that only a small subset of dopamine neurons are specialized for carrying reward-relevant information. Different classes of abusable substances appear to act on this dopamine reward system at different anatomical levels and via different sites of action on or near the dopamine neurons. Activation of the reward system by addictive drugs induces an immediate sense of euphoria or pleasure similar to that obtained through activities that naturally produce rewards such as sexual pleasure. This reward effect, termed positive reinforcement, leads to compulsive drug use.

In support of this hypothesis, basic research has shown that addictive drugs reinforce voluntary drug-taking behavior in humans and laboratory animals (Deneau et al., 1969). The development of techniques for studying the reinforcing effects of cocaine and opiates has allowed researchers to establish and validate laboratory models of critical features of drug addiction—the chronic relapsing behaviors of drug-seeking and drug- taking (Griffiths et al., 1980; Brady and Lukas, 1984). Basic research in laboratory animals has shown that drug-reinforced behaviors are influenced by multiple factors including the pharmacological properties of a drug and its specific neuronal receptors and effector systems, the learned behaviors and cognitions established during repeated episodes of drug use, and the environmental cues that accompany drug-seeking and drug-taking (Griffiths et al., 1980; Young and Herling, 1986; Katz, 1989). Furthermore, evidence is accumulating that the reinforcing effects of cocaine and opiates can be reduced by medications that alter their ability to activate the brain's reward system (e.g., Bergman et al., 1990; Woolverton and Kleven, 1992). In the case of opiates, preclinical studies of methadone, levo-alpha-acetylmethadol (LAAM), naltrexone, and buprenorphine in the reinforcement model have yielded results consistent with those from clinical studies demonstrating the potential effectiveness of these medications as treatment approaches (reviewed by Mello, 1991, 1992). In the case of cocaine, preliminary data suggest a good concordance between results of animal studies in the reinforcement model and preliminary human trials of potential medications (e.g., Fischman et al., 1990; Kosten et al., 1992a). As our understanding of the mechanism of drug addiction continues to improve, development of medications to treat drug addiction will be enhanced.

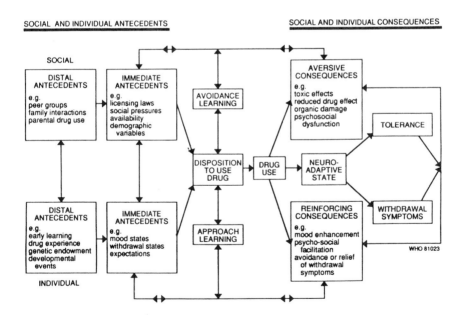

FIGURE 2.1 World Health Organization schematic model of drug use and dependence (Edwards et al., 1981). Figures 2.2 and 2.3 represent modifications and elaborations of Figure 2.1. Reproduced, by permission of WHO.

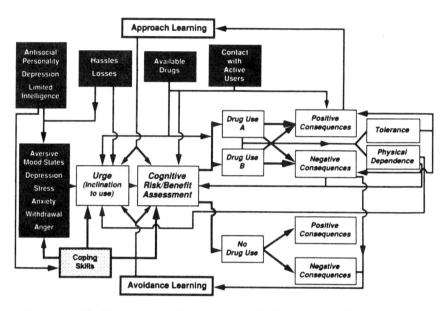

FIGURE 2.2 Modification of the WHO model. This figure is a modification of Figure 2.1 that emphasizes that processes that subserve the urge to use drugs can be distinct from processes that subserve cognitive risk-benefit analysis and that both can be influenced by distinct factors. Note consequences of alternative drug-use or no drug-use decisions and variety of factors shown by recent research to influence mood, urge to use drugs, and capacity (coping skills) to avoid drug use. Reprinted with permission of Raven Press from Jaffe, 1992.

Compulsive drug use is a chronic relapsing disorder, focusing attention on how the behavioral and physiological effects of drugs change over long periods of repeated use. Depending on the particular drug involved and its specific effects, tolerance might develop and be marked (e.g., Fischman et al., 1985). Thus, the user might require increasingly large doses of the drug to obtain the same effects; indeed the initial euphoric effects of a person's first experience with the drug are difficult to reproduce and in some cases are never achieved again. Sensitization can also occur; that is, the person might experience greater effects of the drug at a constant dose. The same drug can produce tolerance to some of its effects and sensitization to others.

Psychological and physical dependence implies that a definable, reproducible, and undesirable withdrawal syndrome will occur if the drug is abruptly stopped. For many addictive drugs, there is a definable acute-abstinence syndrome that is qualitatively and quantitatively different from protracted-abstinence syndrome. Acute abstinence, usually lasting for several days or weeks, is more intense and uncomfortable than protracted abstinence. Protracted abstinence is associated with more subtle symptoms, such as nervousness, insomnia, depression, craving, and vague feelings of discomfort and dysphoria. Symptoms of protracted abstinence can last for months to years and can increase the probability of relapse, a return to the addictive substance. The biological basis of protracted symptoms and craving is virtually unknown. Nevertheless, after extended drug use, withdrawal discomfort or "craving" contributes to sustained, compulsive drug use.

The final stage in the cycle of addiction is relapse. Relapse can occur even after medical treatment of acute withdrawal symptoms and psychosocial treatment for psychological and social problems associated with the addictive disorder. Relapse can be triggered by some of the same factors that initially led to drug use, but it often seems unrelated to the original cause of the drug use. Intelligence, motivation, and high socioeconomic class do not necessarily prevent relapse. Athletes have terminated careers involving millions of dollars in salaries by relapsing to cocaine use.

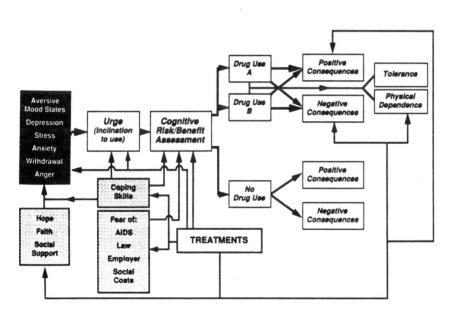

FIGURE 2.3 Model of drug use and dependence including amelioration influences. This figure is a modification of Figure 2.2 that deletes (for visual clarity) some relationships shown in Figures 2.1 and 2.2 and introduces some of the multiple influences (including treatment) that can ameliorate patterns of harmful drug use (including dependence). Reprinted with permission of Raven Press from Jaffe, 1992.

After a person has become addicted to a drug, relapse appears at times to take on an involuntary aspect; this problem has been extensively reviewed (O'Brien et al., 1992). Several categories of variables can contribute to relapse. One factor involves the presence of protracted withdrawal symptoms, most extensively studied in opiate-addicted patients and alcoholics (Martin and Jasinski, 1969). There is some evidence that long-term brain changes occur after chronic cocaine use, and these might be associated with protracted withdrawal symptoms in cocaine addicted individuals (Volkow et al., 1990). Relapse is also associated with the presence of psychiatric disorders in addition to the drug addiction (McLellan et al., 1979; Rounsaville et al., 1982; Khantzian, 1985).

Another class of variables that has been linked to relapse is conditioning factors, that is, environmental factors and physiological states that become associated with each other over time (Wikler, 1973; O'Brien, 1975). Extensive reports show that the rewarding effects of drug use can become associated with particular settings or environments; when formerly addicted patients have been detoxified and treated in a drugfree program, there is an increased probability of relapse to drug use if they are returned to the environment in which they had used drugs (Pratt, 1991). Laboratory studies have demonstrated autonomic nervous system and subjective changes in formerly addicted patients presented with videotaped cues specific to the drugs that they had used (Ehrman et al., 1992). Even highly motivated patients report that these cues produce strong craving for the drug. Accordingly, the use of medications that are effective in reducing the symptoms of protracted abstinence will need to be coupled with behavioral techniques to address conditioned responses.

Addiction is characterized by compulsive drug use, tolerance, dependence, craving, and relapse. Key problems in addiction are: how to prevent the onset of compulsive drug use and how to prevent relapse and the craving that leads to relapse. In the past, much medical attention has been given to treatment (detoxification) for the symptoms of acute abstinence. Acute abstinence syndromes related to a wide array of abused substances can be treated reasonably well with available medications; treatment usually does not even require hospitalization (Hayashida et al., 1989). However, the most difficult problem is preventing relapse to drug use, and relapse prevention is the focal point of much current addiction research, and it is the proper focus of the MDD program. Yet, knowledge about the pathophysiology of the syndromes of protracted abstinence and conditioned withdrawal or relapse is still rudimentary and presents an important challenge to development of anti-addiction medications.

BIOLOGICAL CORRELATES AND
PSYCHOPHARMACOLOGY OF ADDICTION

Opiate Addiction

Opiates can be thought of as a category of plant-derived compounds that happen to activate a major biological system in mammals, the endogenous opiate system. This activation produces many important cardiovascular, endocrine, immune, and neurophysiological effects including euphoria, analgesia, and addiction. Heroin is a well-known example of this group of compounds. These compounds in high doses can produce death from respiratory depression. They also produce abnormalities in the endocrine system that are not easily reversible.

Since the 1960s, it has become clear that the effects of opiate drugs are mediated through interaction with opioid receptors. Moreover, studies of the binding of various related opiate compounds in the brain and other tissues indicate the existence of a multitude of opioid-receptor types and subtypes (Leslie, 1987; Terenius and O'Brien, 1992). The brain contains three major categories of receptors (mu, kappa, and delta), each with at least two subtypes. An opiate drug can simultaneously interact with all three types and act as an agonist (a compound that fully activates a receptor) or partial agonist at each. Binding to the mu receptor, however, is generally considered to be the most important with respect to the pathogenesis of opiate addiction.

The rewarding and subjective effects of opiates are mediated through actions at mu opioid receptors (Holtzman and Locke, 1988; Woods et al., 1988, 1993), and interference with actions at these receptors presents a rational strategy for developing medications for opiate addiction. Specifically, medications that block activation of mu opioid receptors (e.g., naltrexone and long-lasting partial agonists) might reduce drug-taking by preventing or reversing the reinforcing or subjective effects of opiates, whereas medications that produce long-lasting receptor activation and tolerance (e.g., methadone and LAAM) might reduce compulsive drug use by substituting at the receptor site of action and block euphoria and withdrawal (reviewed by Preston and Bigelow, 1991; Mello and Mendelson, 1992). Research examining the effects of opiate maintenance or antagonist treatments on voluntary drug-rewarded behaviors in laboratory animals (e.g., Jones and Prada, 1977; Harrigan and Downs, 1978; Mello et al., 1981) has provided the framework for rational development of medications for opiate addiction (Mello and Mendelson, 1992).

Until very recently, attempts to characterize the opioid receptor at the molecular level had been unsuccessful. However, in 1992 the delta receptor was cloned and sequenced (Evans et al., 1992; Kieffer et al., 1992); the mu and kappa receptors were similarly cloned (Chen et al., 1993a,b; Li et al., 1993; Meng et al., 1993; Wang et al., 1993; Yasuda et al., 1993). It is now possible to express the individual types of receptor in isolated cells, making it easier to characterize their specific properties in detail. Such molecular studies will undoubtedly facilitate the unraveling of some of the complexities of opiate drug use and possibly addiction. They will probably also aid in the further identification and development of agonists and antagonists (compounds that block activation of the receptor) that are specific for an individual type of receptor. In turn, the availability of such selective chemical probes might provide new mechanistic insights that can be applied to the development of medications to treat the various aspects of opiate addiction.

As a result of the identification of the opioid receptors in the early 1970s endogenous ligands (peptides) for the receptor were isolated and characterized. These function as neurotransmitters, neurotransmitter modulators, or neurohormones. Three distinct families of peptides have been identified: enkephalins, endorphins, and dynorphins (Simon and Hiller, 1994). Considerable knowledge has been obtained with respect to the physiological role of the endogenous opiate peptides in normal physiological function. Although the endorphins bind to all three opioid receptor types, they bind preferentially to the mu-receptor, whereas the enkephalins interact with delta and, to a lesser extent, mu receptors, and dynorphins appear to interact with the kappa receptor. Beta-endorphin is present in circulating plasma and appears to function as an endocrine hormone. Its release is therefore coupled with the release of adrenocorticotrophic hormone (ACTH) and melanocyte-stimulating hormone (MSH). The feedback of systemic cortisol and endogenous, as well as exogenous, opiates on the hypothalamus inhibits the release of pro-opiomelanocortin (POMC) peptides. Thus, the function of the hypothalamic-pituitary-adrenal axis is intimately tied to the physiology of the endogenous opiate system. In contrast, the other endogenous opiates seem to have more neurotransmitter or paracrine functions.

Despite the accumulation of considerable knowledge about the impact of opioid-receptor activity on physiological and behavioral functioning, including tolerance and dependence, the molecular mechanisms involved remain to be defined. All opioid receptors appear to be coupled to molecular effector systems involving so-called G-proteins. By analogy to similar types of receptors, it is likely that opiates regulate signaling across cell membranes that requires a complex interplay of molecules including adenylyl cyclase, protein kinases, and various ion channels (K^+, Ca^{2+}) (North, 1979; Crain et al., 1986; Childers, 1991; Harris and Nestler, 1993; Nestler and Greengard, 1994). Presumably, opiate inhibition of adenylyl cyclase results in alterations in the structure (via phosphorylation) of intracellular proteins that change their functioning and account for many of the acute effects of opiates on neuronal function (Nestler, 1992). It appears that adaptations in some of the same intracellular signaling pathways represent part of the molecular basis of opiate tolerance and dependence. Despite considerable progress in recent years (Guitart and Nestler, 1989; Guitart et al.,

1990), much more understanding is required at this mechanistic level before it can be applied to the discovery and development of treatment medications.

Recent information shows that among the many effects of endogenous opiate peptides and opiates on neurons are changes in gene expression. Such alterations in gene expression are presumed to be important in drug addiction because of its gradual and progressive development and the persistence of many of its features long after discontinuation of drug exposure. Studies have demonstrated that opiates can regulate some transcription factors that are important in neuronal gene expression (Chang et al., 1988; Hayward et al., 1990; Guitart et al., 1992; Nestler et al., 1993). That could be important in the long-term adaptations induced by opiates in the brain that ultimately lead to addiction. Many other additional, and poorly understood, adaptive changes probably also contribute to opiate reinforcement, tolerance, and dependence (Nestler, 1992; Nestler et al., 1993).

Work to date suggests that use of opiate drugs can effect long-term changes in the brain that can be successfully treated with medications. Although mu and delta opioid receptors appear to play important roles in the development of opiate tolerance and dependence, it has been difficult to relate reinforcement, tolerance, or dependence to changes in these receptors themselves (Loh and Smith, 1990; Nestler, 1992).

The acute withdrawal of opiates from humans who are tolerant to and dependent on those drugs produces a reproducible physiological syndrome. The syndrome consists of yawning, lacrimation, rhinorrhea, perspiration, mydriasis, tremor, gooseflesh, restlessness, myalgia, anorexia, nausea, vomiting, abdominal cramps, diarrhea, fever, hyperpnea, hypertension, and, if prolonged, weight loss (Kleber, 1981). Many of these acute manifestations of opiate withdrawal represent hyperactivity of the noradrenergic system, thought to be mediated by the loss of opiate feedback inhibition to a specific brain region, the locus ceruleus (Gold et al., 1979; Koob, 1992; Nestler, 1992). The alpha-2-noradrenergic agonist clonidine reduces noradrenergic activity by autoreceptor activation and can ameliorate many of the signs and symptoms of early withdrawal. However, clonidine has proved to be of limited usefulness in the treatment of opiate craving and in the prevention of relapse to addiction (Kleber et al., 1985; Fraser, 1990).

After acute withdrawal of opiates most drug-free formerly addicted patients will still feel uncomfortable. Discomfort can take the form of quantifiable symptoms such as restlessness, irritability, poor concentration, and sleep disturbances which might persist for months or even years (Pratt, 1991). Those symptoms are not relieved by clonidine. Subjects on clonidine might also complain of drug craving and engage in drug-seeking behavior and relapse to drug use. However, methadone, a mu-receptor agonist, is capable of blocking the euphoria of simultaneously administered opiates and inhibiting the symptoms of acute and chronic abstinence, including craving. Its clinical efficacy has been shown to be dose-dependent and enhanced by the provision of ancillary psychosocial services (McLellan et al., 1993).

About 117,000 heroin-addicted individuals in the United States are being treated with methadone and are able to perform normally in the workplace (see Chapter 4 for discussion of the effectiveness of methadone maintenance treatment). An additional benefit of methadone treatment is that it can give opiate-addicted patients, who typically suffer from multiple medical problems, access to other health-care services. A good methadone program can provide medications for infectious diseases and treatment of psychiatric disorders and other clinical problems that often accompany and aggravate opiate-addicted patients' health status.

LAAM, another opiate agonist has recently been approved for use in the treatment of opiate addiction, primarily because of MDD's efforts and those of the Food and Drug Administration (FDA). LAAM is similar to methadone but stays in the body longer and has active metabolites that persist for days, so it can be taken as infrequently as three times per week. For some patients not having to go to a clinic daily for medication removes a major disruption from their lives.

Naltrexone, an antagonist, exploits the specificity of opiate binding to the mu opioid receptor. Naltrexone binds preferentially to the mu receptor and so prevents the binding of any opiate agonist. In animal studies, naltrexone acts to block or reverse the rewarding and subjective effects of mu opiates, and in fact its affinity for the mu receptor is 140 times greater than that of morphine (Holtzman and Locke, 1988; Woods et al., 1993). Naltrexone is being used clinically after detoxification and acute withdrawal to help patients stay off opiate agonist by blocking their effects. Thus, patients taking naltrexone cannot achieve euphoria if they take heroin, so the positive reinforcing effects of opiate addiction are reduced or eliminated (Rose and Levin, 1992). Naltrexone, however, does not relieve all the symptoms of protracted abstinence. In particular, craving, anxiety, and depression are still present, and a person being treated with naltrexone can readily relapse if the naltrexone is stopped. For this reason, naltrexone has proved most valuable in highly motivated addicted patients who have a great socioeconomic risk or other risk associated with relapse, such as medical personnel or parolees. MDD is developing an improved delivery system for naltrexone that would reduce treatment failure due to noncompliance. An implantable "depot" form of naltrexone, for example, that lasts 30–60 days would help a patient who is ambivalent about remaining opiate-free.

Buprenorphine is another new medication for the treatment of opiate addiction. It is a partial mu agonist; i.e., it can mimic the effects of agonists under some conditions (especially conditions in which low doses of agonists are effective) but antagonize effects of agonists under other conditions.

New approaches to medications for opiate addiction might include

• More effective forms of the above medications—for example, agents that selectively interact with the various opioid-receptor subtypes or novel partial agonists that work at the mu opioid receptors.
• A completely new category of medications, such as anticraving compounds to reduce relapse in patients who have been detoxified from opiates.

A wealth of scientific information and understanding of opiate effects, ranging from the clinical to the molecular, has been obtained over the last several decades. This information will continue to grow, especially at the molecular level, primarily through NIDA-supported research. MDD should continue to apply new fundamental knowledge to the study and development of potentially more specific medications for opiate addiction. These might include delta receptor agonists and antagonists or novel partial agonists. At the same time, the clinical evaluation of new medications (such as buprenorphine) or delivery systems (e.g., depot naltrexone) should be continued. Finally, a long-term scientific program should be established with the focus of developing a completely new category of medications based on their anticraving effects.

Cocaine Addiction

Cocaine addiction differs importantly from opiate addiction. Opiates produce an initial calming effect, and dosing takes place two to four times per day. But, cocaine is a stimulant that produces intense, brief euphoria, and dosing typically takes place as often as every 15–30 minutes for hours or even days. Cocaine users tend to use the drug intermittently in binges, rather than in relatively stable daily doses. Cocaine can be taken by several routes; its toxicity depends on its concentrations in the blood and brain. The euphoric effect of cocaine is a function not just of the blood concentration, but of the rapidity and degree of rise of that concentration. The faster the drug reaches the brain, the more euphoric the effect; if the drug is taken intranasally, this takes 90 seconds, intravenously or by smoking 15 seconds (as this involves no dilution with venous blood from the rest of the body).

A major pharmacological effect of cocaine associated with its addictive properties is on the dopaminergic system of the brain (Koob, 1992; Wise and Hoffman, 1992). Specifically, cocaine blocks the reuptake of dopamine in the synaptic cleft by the dopamine transporter. That increases the amount of dopamine available to dopamine receptors and leads to activation of dopaminergic pathways. Although the brain contains several neural pathways rich in dopamine, most attention has focused on the mesolimbic dopamine system for the rewarding actions of cocaine (Kuhar et al., 1991; Koob, 1992; Wise and Hoffman, 1992). Interestingly, the same neural pathway might play a critical role in the reinforcing effects of opiates and most other abused substances.

Recent work has provided information on the molecular basis of acute cocaine action and the dopamine transporter protein has been cloned and sequenced (Amara and Kuhar, 1993). Those results have facilitated a major focus of MDD: to develop drugs with unique binding properties for the dopamine transporter that could serve potentially as cocaine agonists or antagonists.

Similarly, multiple subtypes of dopamine receptors have been identified through molecular cloning (Gingrich and Caron, 1993). All known dopamine receptors, like opioid receptors, are coupled to a G-protein effector system (Duman and Nestler, in press). The D_1 and D_5 receptors produce their effects through the activation of adenylyl cyclase and the cyclic adenosine 3'5'-monophosphate (cyclic AMP) pathway. The D_2, D_3, and D_4 receptors have effects similar to the opioid receptors: they can activate potassium channels, inhibit calcium channels, and inhibit adenylyl cyclase and the cyclic AMP pathway.

Presumably, prolonged blockade of the dopamine transporter results in long-term adaptations in the mesolimbic dopamine system that are responsible for cocaine's addictiveness (Kuhar et al., 1991; Koob, 1992; Nestler, 1992; Wise and Hoffman, 1992). The long-term adaptations are only now beginning to be identified. There is growing evidence that chronic exposure to cocaine can result in impairment of mesolimbic dopamine function (e.g., Brock et al., 1990; Robertson et al., 1991; Weiss et al., 1992), although this remains controversial. Perhaps consistent with such an impairment, some neurons in the mesolimbic dopamine system seem to have increased responsiveness to dopamine signals (Henry and White, 1991). This supersensitivity occurs in the absence of changes in dopamine receptors, but could be explained by adaptations in G-proteins and the cyclic AMP pathway (Nestler, 1992; Nestler et al., 1993). Chronic cocaine use has also been reported recently to produce long-term changes in the expression of the dopamine transporter molecule itself (Cerruti et al., 1994), as well as in specific genetic transcription factors (Young et al., 1991; Hope et al., 1992; Moratalla et al., 1993); these changes could also contribute to the persistent changes that cocaine produces in the brain.

Not every drug that inhibits dopamine uptake produces euphoria or other rewarding effects. Cocaine's effects on the brain reward system might also involve other neurotransmitter systems, for example, those mediated by serotonin and norepinephrine, whose reuptake is inhibited by cocaine (Kuhar et al., 1991) and interactions among these neurotransmitter systems and the endogenous opiate peptide systems are likely. It is still unclear, however, how neurotransmitter systems function and interact in the various aspects of cocaine use and addiction. The potential involvement of such a wide range of neurotransmitter systems in cocaine's actions makes the development of a treatment medication difficult because no single target site is immediately apparent. In fact, an optimal strategy might require the use of several drugs that have different mechanisms of action. Animal researchers have identified specific behavioral effects produced by acute cocaine administration, and have related them to neuropharmacological actions of cocaine at neuronal transporters for the biogenic amines (Fibiger et al., 1992) thereby identifying additional potential targets for medication development.

Abstinence from cocaine use involves complex subjective phenomena that might require medication, but animal models have not yet been developed for these phenomena and could warrant new research investment. During the first 24–48 hours of acute abstinence, cocaine-addicted individuals experience a constellation of symptoms that has been termed "the crash." Early on, they are agitated, depressed, and anorexic and have a strong craving for cocaine. Then they become fatigued, depressed, and somnolent, and that state is followed by exhaustion, hypersomnolence (increased sleeping), and hyperphagia (increased eating). In inpatients, the symptoms gradually resolve over a few days to 2 weeks (Weddington et al., 1990; Satel et al., 1991). In outpatient studies, where cocaine and cues are available, there appears to be a more persistent withdrawal syndrome (Gawin and Kleber, 1986). After the period of acute abstinence has resolved, addicted patients experience prolonged dysphoria that has been termed anergia, depression, anhedonia, or psychasthenia. They have an inability to feel pleasure (anhedonia), and anxiety might accompany this highly subjective symptom complex. Craving occurs separately from anhedonia and is best characterized as a strong memory of the stimulant euphoria. Craving is episodic and can be triggered by changes in mood (positive or negative), geographical location, specific persons or events, or intoxication with other substances (Gawin and Kleber, 1986).

As in opiate addiction, the major clinical problem in treating cocaine addiction is preventing relapse; in contrast, however, effective medications are lacking. Many categories of psychoactive drugs that are already approved for the treatment of various neuropsychiatric disorders, particularly depression, have been tested in clinical trials for cocaine addiction. Tricyclic anti-depressants—specifically desipramine—have decreased the amount of cocaine use in outpatient studies (Gawin et al., 1989), and medications that interfere with cocaine-mediated receptor actions have been shown to alter the rewarding and subjective effects of cocaine in relevant animal models (Spealman, 1992; Woolverton and Kleven, 1992). But no medication is available to clinicians that will consistently reduce the return to cocaine use. As in the treatment of other chronic disorders, the treatment of addiction, including cocaine dependence, must be continued for months or even years to prevent relapse (Brownell et al., 1986).

Scientific understanding of the mechanistic basis of the short-term and long-term addictive affects of cocaine is rudimentary. Recent advances regarding the molecular biology of dopamine transporters and dopaminergic receptors, however, may provide an opportunity for a mechanism-based discovery and development program to be initiated. MDD should continue to use this basic scientific information as it attempts to discover potential medications and not focus exclusively on dopamine receptors and transporters. MDD should also take advantage of the increasing information available on cocaine's neurobiology and molecular mechanism of action in its drug development efforts. The committee acknowledges, however, that the complex mechanisms of cocaine action that result in addiction make the development of a treatment medication difficult and present a major handicap to the development of a rational therapeutic strategy.

MDD AND STRATEGIES FOR THE DISCOVERY OF A COCAINE MEDICATION: DESCRIPTION AND CRITICAL ANALYSIS

Introduction

A medication developed for the treatment of drug addiction ideally is effective when administered orally or is able to be implanted, is long-acting, clinically safe, causes few side effects, is acceptable to patients, is designed to reduce both reinforcing and toxic effects of the addictive drug, has little abuse liability and is useful for more than one class of abused drugs (because many drug-users use more than one drug).

On the basis of the methadone experience, it is reasonable to conclude that effective medications for the treatment of cocaine addiction could reduce the strong tendency of patients to relapse to compulsive cocaine use. What is not clear is whether the strategies that led to methadone and LAAM will be the best strategies for finding medications useful in treating cocaine addiction. For example, methadone was found effective in clinical situations, and animal models were developed that mirrored methadone's effects as a screening test for new compounds such as LAAM. But no such medication exists for cocaine addiction, so there is no way to validate any of the existing and potential animal models that are critical in the screening and initial evaluation of putative drug candidates. The sparseness of the scientific knowledge on cocaine's actions adds to the difficulty in medication development because it is not clear whether the best pharmacological treatment strategy is to target the pleasure-seeking aspect of cocaine use or the dysphoria and distressful consequences of abstinence. Accordingly, approaches directed toward both aspects need to be pursued.

MDD has focused attention on specific classes of drugs in both its opiate-treatment and cocaine-treatment discovery programs. Chemicals belonging to those classes are given high priority for entry into the screening programs. The classes, most of which are aimed at cocaine treatment discovery, are listed below:

- Dopamine-receptor antagonists.
- Dopamine-receptor agonists.
- Opioid-receptor antagonists.
- Opioid-receptor agonists.
- Monoamine-transporter agonists.
- Serotonin-receptor agonists.
- Serotonin-receptor antagonists.
- Antimanic agents.

Source of Compounds

As noted previously in this chapter, a sound and rational scientific basis for the selection of candidate compounds for cocaine addiction does not yet exist. Yet, a source and supply of candidate compounds that can initially be screened for potential activity are critical, as promising compounds can then be used as leads for investigation. MDD may obtain compounds from several sources, including the academic community and chemical supply houses, but the vast majority of compounds are in the chemical libraries of pharmaceutical companies.

MDD has initiated contacts with a number of pharmaceutical companies to obtain compounds for its screening program (described in detail in the next section of this chapter). However, experience in eliciting pharmaceutical industry cooperation with the program has been disappointing (Grudzinskas, 1993; Vocci, 1993). Only about 125 chemicals were provided to MDD by pharmaceutical companies in 1990–1993. MDD representatives feel that the screening program will have to be cut back (Grudzinskas, 1993) if sufficient numbers of compounds are not obtained, with obvious long-term consequences for the ultimate goal of discovering new, potentially active compounds to treat addiction. The reasons for the apparent reluctance of pharmaceutical companies to supply compounds to the MDD for their screening program are discussed in Chapter 3.

A second source of compounds to the MDD is from already marketed drugs or in new psychoactive drugs under development for other indications. In general, many drugs are found to have additional and therapeutically useful effects beyond those for which they are originally approved by FDA. During clinical trials or during treatment (with approved medications), clinicians may notice unexpected benefits in their addicted patients from medications not specifically developed to treat addictions. For example, clonidine, marketed primarily as an antihypertensive agent, was found to be clinically useful for treating opiate withdrawal. Thus, new chemical entities developed by the pharmaceutical industry and having psychopharmacological activity are potential candidates for controlled clinical evaluation in the treatment of cocaine addiction.

While MDD accepts many types of compounds as sources for the cocaine screening program, guidelines for the types of compounds it is seeking have not been clearly articulated. That may result in wasted time, effort and resources.

The committee recommends that MDD develop clear, goal-oriented guidelines for the selection of candidate compounds, that do not depend as heavily on the opiate model. Such guidelines could reduce redundant testing of chemicals with similar pharmacologic profiles. In addition, the committee recommends that MDD increase its consideration of compounds with novel characteristics.

A dramatically different approach might also achieve the desired goal, e.g., the discovery of an anticraving compound or the application of biotechnology products, such as monoclonal antibodies. Recent basic research has shown that some monoclonal catalytic antibodies can cleave cocaine at the benzoylecgonine moiety rendering it inactive and at the same time regenerate their hydrolytic activity (Landry et al., 1993). The antibody (or other ways of neutralizing cocaine directly) has the advantage that the essential dopamine system is left intact and functional. This type of research is perhaps an example of the kind of innovative approach that MDD should identify and pursue aggressively.

Medication Preclinical Screening

Given the absence of a mechanism of action or a "lead" compound for the treatment of cocaine addiction, MDD established the Cocaine Treatment Discovery Program (CTDP) (Chapter 3). Chemicals are accepted into CTDP screening if they have CNS activity and are likely to have direct or indirect biochemical interactions with dopamine or serotonin. Once a chemical has been identified and accepted for preclinical screening, the protocol used depends on what is known about it. CTDP has developed a tiered strategy that can use both in vitro biochemical assays and in vivo behavioral tests (Figure 2.4). Screening of chemicals that are known to affect the dopamine system and have CNS activity can begin with in vivo behavioral testing rather than in vitro testing. Ultimately, the CTDP hopes to identify promising candidates for further toxicological and human clinical testing.

This section examines MDD's CTDP and assesses this program according to established methods of chemical identification and behavioral pharmacology. As noted, once a chemical is identified as a potential drug candidate, it undergoes in vitro or in vivo screening.

In Vitro Screen—Receptors and Mechanisms of Action

One strategy used by MDD to find chemicals that bind to a cocaine receptor is mechanism-based (Figure 2.4). Chemicals are subjected to a battery of in vitro biochemical assays to see whether they prevent cocaine from binding without producing effects of their own on the transporter's function. That approach could provide acute cocaine blocking agents analogous to naltrexone. The recent cloning and expression of the relevant transporter proteins make it possible to determine readily whether a so-called cocaine blocker is feasible. This could be accomplished in a more targeted way by combining the knowledge of the structures of chemicals with yet to be obtained information on the structures of the transporter proteins, as opposed to experimental screening of large numbers of potential drug candidates.

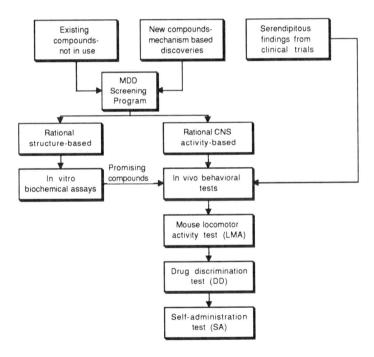

FIGURE 2.4 Cocaine treatment screening flowchart. MDD's CTDP screening program analyzes compounds from industry, academia, or other sources through a series of assays including in vitro biochemical assays or in vivo behavioral assays. Compounds found serendipitously in clinical trials to be potentially useful for treating cocaine addiction are put through the in vivo screens to test the validity of the screens.

The mechanism-based approach, however, has potential flaws: not all of cocaine's immediate stimulatory effects on the brain are mediated by dopaminergic mechanisms. In addition, other drugs that produce behavioral effects similar to those of cocaine, such as amphetamines, have different mechanisms of action, such as increased release of monoamines from nerve terminals (Cooper et al., 1991). A cocaine-blocker would be expected to have no effect on the action of such other stimulants so that treated patients might simply abuse other stimulants while using a cocaine-blocker. That possibility is supported by the fact that polydrug abuse and substituting and experimenting with available drugs are the rule, rather than the exception, for drug users. In addition, it is not known whether the blockade of the dopamine transporter can be achieved without affecting its functioning with regard to dopamine, which is critical in normal neurotransmission.

To overcome such obstacles, MDD has emphasized the development of potential antagonists that interact with the dopamine receptor itself, because the antagonists would be expected to block many of the acute effects of cocaine and other stimulants. There is, however, considerable clinical evidence of the lack of utility of current nonselective dopamine antagonists in the treatment of cocaine addition. Accordingly, MDD is now trying to develop drugs with increasing specificity (i.e., selective for each of the known dopamine-receptor subtypes). This approach is based on the assumption that increased selectivity will be associated with increased effectiveness—an assumption that is largely untested. Indeed, some of the most widely used and effective drugs (e.g., aspirin, lithium, and benzodiazepines) have the least-specific mechanisms of action.

The obstacles outlined above underscore the complexity of the issues involved in developing medications for cocaine addiction. The effects on the dopamine system will have to be characterized for any compound eventually used to treat cocaine addiction, and compounds that act on the dopamine system may actually be found to be effective when administered in combination with compounds with activity in non-dopamine systems. Although the focus on the dopamine system presents problems, no other neurotransmitter system seems a more attractive target. Unlike drug design for opiate addiction, there is no current medication that is effective in treating cocaine addiction. If such a medication existed, its mechanism of action would provide a tremendously useful basis for development of new screening strategies.

In Vivo Screen—Behavioral Tests

The other component of CTDP consists of a sequence of animal behavioral tests for studying potential cocaine-treatment medications. Three assays are used in this order: the locomotor-activity (LMA) test, the drug-discrimination (DD) test, and the self-administration (SA) test. Each initially uses rodents (mice or rats); promising compounds are then tested in monkeys. The goal of the behavioral component of the screening program—which, like the physiological tests, draws on NIDA-sponsored basic research—is to identify compounds with the potential to interfere with or mimic the rewarding effects of cocaine but without abusive, toxic, or rewarding effects of their own. Compounds that mimic some of cocaine's actions might serve as replacement or substitution therapies, whereas compounds that antagonize cocaine might be used to block the effects of cocaine after a relapse to use.

The LMA test is based on the knowledge that cocaine increases locomotor activity in mice. A compound that increases such activity when administered alone might substitute for cocaine (agonist effects). A compound that does not increase this activity, might have no useful effect or might actually block cocaine's actions (antagonist effects). On the basis of results of the LMA test, potential antagonist compounds are tested with cocaine to see whether they block cocaine-induced increases in locomotor activity. Potential agonists are tested with cocaine to see if they have partial agonist effects that will block those of cocaine.

Results of LMA tests constitute the major decision point regarding further screening of a chemical (Figure 2.4). The next step is to assess whether the chemical can substitute for cocaine in (DD) tests or block cocaine's discriminative properties.[1] Discriminative stimulus effects of drugs in laboratory animals are pharmacologically specific and are often predictive of subjective effects in humans (Johanson, 1992; Preston and Bigelow, 1991). Moreover, the high correlation of discriminative effects with neuropharmacological actions of drugs allows exploration of the neuropharmacological mechanisms that underlie the subjective effects of cocaine.

The SA test is a direct test of the rewarding effects of drugs. It has been noted that animals will consistently self-administer cocaine, often to the exclusion of food or other reinforcers. Thus, a test chemical that blocks cocaine self-administration might be useful in treating cocaine addiction. That chemical, however, might also be avidly self-administered and thus have abuse potential; such chemicals are tested further without cocaine to assess that possibility. Eventually, promising chemicals are tested in all the tests outlined above, and the resulting information is used as baseline data for further development.

MDD moved rapidly to select and implement three behavioral models for initial screening of candidate chemicals. On the basis of available scientific

---

[1]Discriminative properties of a drug encompass all possible perceived and physiological effects of the drug. To be effective, a "substitute" drug, even if it may not produce all the effects of the drug of interest, will produce a sufficient number to reduce or eliminate use of the original drug. Buprenorphine is a good example of such a substitute in the opioid system.

knowledge about the behavioral and neuropharmacological effects of cocaine, those models were reasonable first choices. In particular, the models selected have been well characterized pharmacologically and behaviorally (Griffiths et al., 1980; Colpaert and Balster, 1988; Spealman et al., 1992).

Specific Conclusions and Recommendations for the MDD

At this early date, it is difficult to assess the progress of the screening protocols. The effectiveness of the protocols and their predictive value in humans might be seriously limited, however, because of

- The lack of knowledge on the mechanism of cocaine addiction.
- The lack of animal models for addiction, craving, and relapse.
- The lack of successful treatments in humans against which animal models could be validated.
- The lack of potentially useful chemicals from industry, academe, etc.
- The acute administration of candidate chemicals during screening, whereas anti-addiction medications will be clinically administered over time.

The committee recommends that MDD critically evaluate the usefulness of its preclinical screen for discovery of medications to treat cocaine addiction, inasmuch as current methods may not be predictive for humans.

MDD should provide clear guidance to researchers based on results of molecular, cellular and behavioral studies.

MDD should evaluate alternative biochemical targets, such as nondopaminergic mechanisms and the growing number of postreceptor proteins implicated in cocaine's actions.

MDD should explore new ways to seek continuing scientific guidance from intramural and extramural researchers regarding management and refinement of its preclinical screening procedures (as the committee is aware of budgetary and hiring constraints placed on NIDA).

Clinical Trials

In the absence of a clear understanding of the complexity of cocaine's effects on the brain and lack of candidate compounds, there is an alternative approach to identifying potentially useful medications for cocaine addiction: evaluation of the efficacy of currently available psychopharmacological agents to treat the various aspects of cocaine addiction. A number of drugs, approved for indications other than treating drug addiction, have been clinically investigated over the last several years. Many of these investigations have been investigator-initiated and spontaneous (not necessarily funded by NIDA).

That strategy was taken with gepirone, a drug that facilitates serotonin neurotransmission in the brain, and bupropion, an antidepressant with stimulant properties. The findings were negative for both compounds. They were tested initially in multiclinic trials, however, if gepirone and bupropion had first been evaluated in more moderate-sized double-blinded trials, resources could have been saved and the multiclinic strategy reserved for more promising medications.

Unfortunately, the typical history has been that open clinical trials of potential medications have shown apparent effects but there has been failure to confirm such effects consistently in carefully controlled studies. Even agents that show effectiveness in double blind studies (e.g., desipramine in Gawin et al., 1989) might not be effective for different populations such as cocaine-using methadone patients, unless subpopulations are carefully analyzed; e.g., desipramine showed effectiveness in the methadone studies if antisocial-personality patients were removed from the analysis (Arndt et al., 1992; Arndt et al., in press; Kosten et al., 1992b; Leal et al., in press).

The committee believes, however, that studies should be designed to take full advantage of serendipity. The study design is critical; nonblinded and uncontrolled studies should be avoided (Fraser, 1990). Randomized controlled trials with enough patients to ensure adequate statistical power are preferred. The process by which subjects are selected for study should control for confounding variables such as polydrug use; 20 percent of cocaine users self-medicate the cocaine crash with ethanol; 50 percent of opiate users also use cocaine, and psychiatric comorbidity must be controlled for because cocaine-addicted patients with other diagnoses especially attention deficit disorder, major depression, and bipolar disorders—respond differently to different medications (Metzger et al., 1989). In addition, studies that include subjective ratings of craving should be confirmed objectively, with a urine screen.

The committee believes that candidate compounds should be tested in rigorously controlled, moderate-size trials and in a limited number of sites; promising compounds can then be further evaluated in multi-clinic settings.

It has been shown that statistically significant results can often be achieved when 20 to 30 individuals participate in a clinical trial in both the test and placebo controlled groups (Alterman et al., 1992). While the committee acknowledges that the power analysis indicates that small effects will be missed, they nonetheless believe that the ability to screen more substances for substantial effects, with the given resources, is worth the risk of missing small effects.

Not only would that approach save resources, but moderate-sized studies can often answer the questions being posed by the larger, multiclinic studies more quickly. Finally, selection of compounds based on a systematic analysis of chemical structure would be advantageous before selection of drugs for clinical evaluation. Promising candidates might also be initially evaluated with appropriate laboratory methods (Fischman and Foltin, 1992). MDD's focus on evaluating multiple members of the same classes of compounds might be questionable and could result in nonproductive, resource-intensive efforts for many years.

The clinical evaluation of promising medications, whether derived from screening procedures or from the armamentarium of currently approved drugs, is resource-intensive, and the validity of the findings depends heavily on appropriate experimental design.

Human Behavioral Models

Two test models that have been developed in human subjects are used to screen potential medications for their efficacy in the treatment of cocaine addiction (Fischman and Foltin, 1992; Robbins et al., 1992). These tests are conducted in the laboratory and are completed more rapidly than long-term clinical trials. They have not yet been sufficiently validated as to their predictive potential for determining medications that are likely to be effective in clinical trials.

In the first model, volunteers are given the opportunity to take repeated doses of cocaine, with doses and patterning approximating those reported in natural settings (Fischman and Foltin, 1992). Separate measures are made of the amount of drug taken, cardiovascular effects, subjective effects, and craving. The results can be compared with the results measured when the volunteers are given potential treatment medications. In addition, volunteers are given the opportunity to choose between cocaine and nondrugs (a similarity to the ordinary setting, where alternative reinforcers are available); this allows the investigator to determine how medications might interact with other behavioral treatment approaches (Fischman and Foltin, 1992).

The second model evaluates human subjects' responses to cocaine-related cues (Robbins et al., 1992). It relies on the conditioned effects of long-term cocaine use. It has been noted that after detoxification cocaine-addicted patients with the determination to refrain from further cocaine use, regardless of the form of psychotherapy, are likely to experience involuntary reactions (such as cocaine craving and other psychological changes) when they return to areas in which they previously used cocaine. Those reactions can also be produced by videotape or other stimuli associated with cocaine even when presented to drugfree former cocaine-addicted patients in the laboratory. A medication that dampens these cue-elicited responses might have a protective value in the enhancement of cocaine-treatment programs.

Theoretically, a large number of compounds could be screened with the two models, and those which seem to dampen drug-taking or the craving response could be studied in clinical trials that are more time-consuming and costly.

CONCLUSIONS AND RECOMMENDATIONS

The initiation and maintenance of drug addiction are complex, involving psychologic, physiologic, interpersonal, and social variables. Of particular focus in the MDD program is development of refined medications to treat opiate-addicted patients and the discovery of compounds that will be effective in treating cocaine-addicted patients. The concept of using medications to help to treat drug-addicted individuals is based on the physiological correlates of drug addiction, and the strategy has been shown to be extremely useful as part of the treatment of opiate addiction. Development of effective medications, however, depends heavily on an adequate knowledge base derived from basic scientific studies. Although the science base for opiates is rich, there are large gaps in knowledge about cocaine. In addition, patterns of cocaine use differ greatly from patterns of opiate use and the differences must be taken into account in understanding the physiological underpinnings of the use of these drugs. The largest gaps are related to craving, which likely represents the most important factor in relapse to drug use once an addict is detoxified and enters treatment.

Emerging evidence suggests that chronic administration of both opiates and cocaine produces adaptive responses in numerous behavioral and physiological systems. Research on tolerance and sensitization suggests that chronic drug use can change the neuronal systems with which addictive drugs interact, but only rudimentary information is available on the cellular and molecular bases of these changes for either opiates or cocaine. Moreover, treatment medications themselves can have different effects in acute or repeated administration, and relatively little is known about how chronic treatment with a medication can alter the subjective or voluntary components of addiction. For those reasons, the committee believes that it is imperative to foster NIDA's basic research efforts in the mechanism of cocaine addiction and in the molecular, cellular, and behavioral bases of chronic drug effects. Basic research to develop laboratory models of critical behavioral characteristics of the addictive process is also needed.

Current clinical understanding of the addictive process suggests that models of drug-craving and relapse can be particularly important for medication development. Animal studies exploring such processes as conditioned-stimulus control of drug taking, incentive and motivational effects, and priming effects have begun to identify potential targets for treatment medications. Identification of such behavioral models must be followed by extensive pharmacological and behavioral characterization to provide benchmarks for evaluation of potential medications. A basic understanding of "craving" is also needed at both the clinical and preclinical levels. Therefore, the committee strongly believes that unless basic research is supported at an appropriate funding level, it will be difficult to make important progress in the scientific knowledge base. The lack of such knowledge would continue to hamper the private sector and MDD in the development of a medication.

In relation specifically to MDD, the committee recommends two mechanisms to address the critical issue of supporting basic science:

The committee recommends that MDD be given a high priority for funding. Although MDD was authorized at $95 million in FY 1994, its appropriation of $40 million has fallen far short of this mark and is far below what is needed for research and development.

The committee is aware, however, of the budget constraints on the institutes of the National Institutes of Health (NIH); as a possible mechanism for increased support, the committee suggests the use of funds from the Special Forfeiture Fund in the Office of National Drug Control Policy (ONDCP).[2] Utilizing a

---

[2]The ONDCP Special Forfeiture Fund results from the transfer of money from the Federal Asset Forfeiture Fund (described below). In FY 1990, the Federal Assets Forfeiture Fund transferred $117 million to federal law-enforcement agencies. Deposits of $17 million were also made to the Special Forfeiture Fund to supplement ONDCP program resources and of $115 million to support Federal prison construction. The use of the Special Forfeiture Fund is at the discretion of the director of ONDCP.

The Federal Asset Forfeiture Fund is a sum of money resulting from the sale of assets used in criminal activity that have been seized by the government. In 1990 DEA seized assets valued at more than $1 billion. About two-fifths of the assets seized by DEA was currency valued at almost $364 million. In addition, DEA seized $346 million worth of real property, 5,674 vehicles worth over $60 million, 187 vessels valued at over $16 million, and 51 airplanes worth over $25 million. Almost two-thirds of DEA's seizures during 1990 resulted from cocaine investigations. DEA seizures that were ultimately forfeited are valued at more than $427 million in 1990 (BJS, 1992).

portion of those funds for basic research not only would provide additional money to MDD, but would demonstrate executive-branch support.

> **The committee recommends that NIDA designate national drug abuse research centers, subject to congressional appropriations, as described in the ADAMHA Reorganization Act [Public Law 102-321, Section 464N (a)], "for the purpose of interdisciplinary research relating to drug abuse and other biomedical, behavioral, and social issues related to drug abuse." These centers would be engaged in and would coordinate all aspects of drug-abuse research, treatment, and education.**

The committee intends that the designation of such centers would serve as focal points for all aspects of drug-abuse research and would have the added benefit of encouraging new investigators to enter the field; they would also serve as sites for clinical trials and for training clinicians (see Chapter 6 for additional text and recommendations on comprehensive centers). The characteristics of the centers should include the conduct of basic research, clinical research, high-priority clinical trial research, and other applied research, drug abuse prevention, training, information, and community service and outreach. One possible mechanism for funding the centers could be through the use of core grants (similar to those used by the National Cancer Institute) because they are designed to bring together an institution's research efforts into a single administrative structure. The grant provides funds for the operation of a centralized administrative staff, resources, and services. It may also provide funding for newly recruited investigators or investigators who have not previously been supported by grants (Chapter 6). By using the core grant mechanism the centers would have the flexibility to explore new research leads. The core grants are not directly designed to support laboratory and clinical research, but they do so indirectly. Alternative funding mechanisms might include the use of contracts, CRADAs, or cooperative agreements between NIDA and the designated center. It should be noted that NIDA does have a number of specialized research centers, but they are more narrowly focused and lack the flexibility of the centers suggested here.

With the designation of such centers, the committee believes that progress will be made in basic, clinical, and other applied research in and treatment of drug addiction. Furthermore, the paucity of basic knowledge in this field is best approached through the coordinated effort that the centers are likely to achieve.

68   DEVELOPMENT OF MEDICATIONS

REFERENCES

Alterman AI, Droba M, Antelo RE, Cornish JW, Sweeney KK, Parikh GA, O'Brien CP. 1992. Amantadine may facilitate detoxification of cocaine addicts. Drug and Alcohol Dependence 31:19–29.

Amara SG, Kuhar MJ. 1993. Neurotransmitter transporters: recent progress. Annual Review of Neuroscience 16:73–93.

APA (American Psychiatric Association). 1987. Diagnostic and Statistical Manual of Mental Disorders, 3rd ed. revised (DSM-III-R). Washington, DC: American Psychiatric Association.

Arndt IO, Dorozynsky L, Woody GE, McLellan AT, O'Brien CP. 1992. Desipramine treatment of cocaine dependence in methadone-maintained patients. Archives of General Psychiatry 49:888–893.

Arndt IO, et al. In press. Desipramine treatment for cocaine dependence: role of antisocial personality disorder. Journal of Nervous and Mental Disease.

Bergman, J, Kamien JB, Spealman RD. 1990. Antagonism of cocaine self-administration by selective dopamine D_1 and D_2 antagonists. Behavioral Pharmacology 1:355–363.

BJS (Bureau of Justice Statistics). 1992. Drugs, Crime, and the Justice System. Washington, DC: Government Printing Office. NCJ-1335652.

Brady JV, Lukas SE, eds. 1984. Testing Drugs for Physical Dependence Potential and Abuse Liability. NIDA Research Monograph 52. DHHS Publication No. (ADM) 87-1332. Washington, DC: U.S. Government Printing Office.

Brock JW, Ng JP, Justice JB Jr. 1990. Effect of chronic cocaine on dopamine synthesis in the nucleus accumbens as determined by microdialysis perfusion with NSD-1015. Neuroscience Letters 117:234–239.

Brownell KD, Marlatt GA, Lichtenstein E, Wilson GT. 1986. Understanding and preventing relapse. American Psychologist 41:765–782.

Cerruti C, Pilotte NS, Uhl G, Kuhar MJ. 1994. Reduction in dopamine transporter MRNA after cessation of repeated cocaine administration. Brain Research: Molecular Brain Research 22:132–138.

Chang SL, Squinto SP, Harlan RE. 1988. Morphine activation of c-fos expression in rat brain. Biochemical and Biophysical Research Communications 157:698–704.

Chen Y, Mestek A, Liu J, Hurley JA, Yu L. 1993a. Molecular cloning and functional expression of a mu-opioid receptor from rat brain. Molecular Pharmacology 44:8–12.

Chen Y, Mestek A, Liu J, Yu L. 1993b. Molecular cloning of a rat kappa-opioid receptor reveals sequence similarities to the mu-opioid and delta-opioid receptors. Biochemical Journal 295:625–628.

Childers SR. 1991. Opioid receptor-coupled second messenger systems. Life Sciences 48:1991–2003.

Colpaert FC, Balster RL, eds. 1988. Transduction Mechanisms of Drug Stimuli. Berlin: Springer-Verlag.

Cooper JR, Bloom FE, Roth RH. 1991. The Biochemical Basis of Neuropharmacology, 6th ed. New York: Oxford University Press.

Crain SM, Crain B, Peterson ER. 1986. Cyclic AMP or forskolin rapidly attenuates the depressant effects of opioids on sensory-evoked dorsal-horn responses in mouse spinal cord-ganglion explants. Brain Research 370:61–72.

Deneau G, Yanagita T, Seevers MH. 1969. Self-administration of psychoactive substances by the monkey. Psychopharmacologia 16:30–48.

Duman RS, Nestler EJ. In press. Signal transduction pathways for catecholamine receptors. In: Bloom FE, Kupfer D, eds. Psychopharmacology: Fourth Generation of Progress. New York: Raven Press.

Edwards G, Arif A, Hodgson R. 1981. Nomenclature and classification of drug- and alcohol-related problems: a WHO memorandum. Bulletin of the World Health Organization 59:225–242.

Ehrman R, Robbins SJ, Childress AR, O'Brien CP. 1992. Conditioned responses to cocaine-related stimuli in cocaine abuse patients. Psychopharmacology 107:523–529.

Evans CJ, Keith DE Jr, Morrison H, Magendzo K, Edwards RH. 1992. Cloning of a delta opioid receptor by functional expression. Science 258:1952–1955.

Fibiger HC, Phillips AG, Brown EE. 1992. The neurobiology of cocaine-induced reinforcement. In: Cocaine: Scientific and Social Dimensions. CIBA Foundation Symposium 166. Chichester: John Wiley. 96–110.

Fischman MW, Foltin RW. 1992. Cocaine: Scientific and Social Dimensions. New York: John Wiley.

Fischman MW, Schuster CR, Javaid J, Hatano Y, Davis J. 1985. Acute tolerance development to the cardiovascular and subjective effects of cocaine. Journal of Pharmacology and Experimental Therapeutics. 235:677–82.

Fischman MW, Foltin RW, Nestadt G, Pearlson GD. 1990. Effects of desipramine maintenance on cocaine self-administration by humans. Journal of Pharmacology and Experimental Therapeutics 253:760–770.

Fraser AD. 1990. Clinical toxicology of drugs used in the treatment of opiate dependency. Clinics in Laboratory Medicine 10:375–386.

Gawin FH, Kleber HD. 1986. Abstinence symptomatology and psychiatric diagnosis in cocaine abusers. Archives of General Psychiatry 43:107–113.

Gawin FH, Kleber HD, Byck R, Rounsaville BJ, Kosten TR, Jatlow PI, Morgan C. 1989. Desipramine facilitation of initial cocaine abstinence. Archives of General Psychiatry 46:117–121.

Gingrich JA, Caron MG. 1993. Recent advances in the molecular biology of dopamine receptors. Annual Review of Neuroscience 16:299–321.

Gold MS, Redmond DE , Kleber HD. 1979. Noradrenergic hyperactivity in opiate withdrawal supported by clonidine reversal of opiate withdrawal. American Journal of Psychiatry. 136:100–102.

Griffiths RR, Bigelow GE, Henningfield JE. 1980. Similarities in animal and human drug-taking behavior. Advances in Substance Abuse 1:1–90.

Grudzinskas CV. 1993. Letter to G. Mossinghoff, President, Pharmaceutical Manufacturers Association. November 10, 1993.

Guitart X, Nestler EJ. 1989. Identification of morphine- and cyclic AMP-regulated phosphoproteins (MARPPs) in the locus coeruleus and other regions of the rat brain: regulation by acute and chronic morphine. Journal of Neuroscience 9:4371–4387.

Guitart X, Hayward M, Nisenbaum LK, Beitner-Johnson DB, Haycock JW, Nestler EJ. 1990. Identification of MARPP-58, a morphine- and cyclic AMP-regulated phosphoprotein of 58 kDa, as tyrosine hydroxylase: evidence for regulation of its expression by chronic morphine in the rat locus coeruleus. Journal of Neuroscience 10:2649–2659.

Guitart X, Thompson MA, Mirante CK, Greenberg ME, Nestler EJ. 1992. Regulation of cyclic AMP response element-binding protein (CREB) phosphorylation by acute and chronic morphine in the rat locus coeruleus. Journal of Neurochemistry 58:1168–1171.

Harrigan SE, Downs DA. 1978. Continuous intravenous naltrexone effects on morphine self-administration in rhesus monkeys. Journal of Pharmacology and Experimental Therapeutics 204:481–486.

Harris HW, Nestler EJ. 1993. Opiate regulation of signal-transduction pathways. In: Hammer RP Jr, ed. The Neurobiology of Opiates. Boca Raton, FL: CRC Press.

Hayashida M, Alterman AI, McLellan AT, O'Brien CP, Purtill JJ, Volpicelli J, Raphaelson AH, Hall CP. 1989. Comparative effectiveness and costs of inpatient and outpatient detoxification of patients with mild to moderate alcohol withdrawal syndrome. New England Journal of Medicine 320:358–365.

Hayward MD, Duman RS, Nestler EJ. 1990. Induction of the c-fos proto-oncogene during opiate withdrawal in the locus coeruleus and other regions of rat brain. Brain Research 525:256–266.

Henry DJ, White FJ. 1991. Repeated cocaine administration causes persistent enhancement of D1 dopamine receptor sensitivity within the rat nucleus accumbens. Journal of Pharmacology and Experimental Therapeutics 258:882–890.

Holtzman SG, Locke KW. 1988. Neural mechanisms of drug stimuli: experimental approaches. In: Colpaert FC, Balster RL, eds. Transduction Mechanisms of Drug Stimuli. Berlin: Springer-Verlag. 139–153.

Hope BT, Kosofsky B, Hyman SE, Nestler EJ. 1992. Regulation of immediate early gene expression and AP-1 binding in the rat nucleus accumbens by chronic cocaine. Proceedings of the National Academy of Sciences (USA) 89:5764–5768.

Jaffe JH. 1992. Current concepts of addiction. In: O'Brien CP, Jaffe JH, eds. Addictive States. New York: Raven Press. 1–21.

Johanson CE. 1992. The use of human drug discrimination studies in medication development. NIDA Research Monograph 119:180–184.

Jones BE, Prada JA. 1977. Effects of methadone and morphine maintenance on drug-seeking behavior in the dog. Psychopharmacology 54:109–112.

Katz JL. 1989. Drugs as reinforcers: pharmacological and behavioural factors. In: Liebman JM, Cooper SJ, eds. The Neuropharmacological Basis of Reward. Oxford: Oxford University Press. 164–213.

Khantzian EJ. 1985. The self-medication hypothesis of addictive disorders: focus on heroin and cocaine dependence. American Journal of Psychiatry 142:1259–1264.

Kieffer BL, Befort K, Gaveriaux-Ruff C, Hirth CG. 1992. The delta-opioid receptor: isolation of a cDNA by expression cloning and pharmacological characterization. Proceedings of the National Academy of Sciences (USA) 89:12048–12052.

Kleber HD. 1981. Detoxification from narcotics. In: Lowinson JH, Ruiz P, eds. Substance Abuse: Clinical Problems and Perspectives. Baltimore: Williams and Wilkins.

Kleber HD, Riordan CE, Rounsaville B, Kosten T, Charney D, Gaspari J, Hogan I, O'Connor C. 1985. Clonidine in outpatient detoxification from methadone maintenance. Archives of General Psychiatry 42:391–394.

Koob GF. 1992. Drugs of abuse: anatomy, pharmacology and function of reward pathways. Trends in Pharmacological Sciences 13:177–184.

Kosten TR, Rosen MI, Schottenfeld R, Ziedonis D. 1992a. Buprenorphine for cocaine and opiate dependence. Psychopharmacology Bulletin 28:15–19.

Kosten TR, Morgan CM, Falcione J, Schottenfeld RS. 1992b. Pharmacotherapy for cocaine-abusing methadone-maintained patients using amantadine or desipramine. Archives of General Psychiatry. 49:894–898.

Kuhar MJ, Ritz MC, Boja JW. 1991. The dopamine hypothesis of the reinforcing properties of cocaine. Trends in Neuroscience 14:299–302.

Landry DW, Zhao K, Yang GX, Glickman M, Georgiadis TM. 1993. Antibody-catalyzed degradation of cocaine Science 259:1899–1901.

Leal J, Ziedonis D, Kosten T. In press. Antisocial personality disorder as a prognostic factor for pharmacotherapy of cocaine dependence. Drug and Alcohol Dependence.

Leslie FM. 1987. Methods used for the study of opioid receptors. Pharmacological Reviews 39:197–249.

Li S, Zhu J, Chen C, Chen YW, Deriel JK, Ashby B, Liu-Chen LY. 1993. Molecular cloning and expression of a rat kappa-opioid receptor. Biochemical Journal 295:629–634.

Loh HH, Smith AP. 1990. Molecular characterization of opioid receptors. Annual Review of Pharmacology and Toxicology 30:123–147.

Martin WR, Jasinski DR. 1969. Physiological parameters of morphine in man: tolerance, early abstinence, protracted abstinence. Journal of Psychiatric Research 7:9–17.

McLellan AT, Woody GE, O'Brien CP. 1979. Development of psychiatric illness in drug abusers. New England Journal of Medicine 301:1310–1314.

McLellan AT, Arndt IO, Metzger DS, Woody GE, O'Brien CP. 1993. The effects of psychosocial services in substance abuse treatment. Journal of the American Medical Association 269:1953–1959.

Mello NK. 1991. Preclinical evaluation of the effects of buprenorphine, naltrexone and desipramine on cocaine self-administration. NIDA Research Monographs 105:189–195.

Mello NK. 1992. Behavioral strategies for the evaluation of new pharmacotherapies for drug abuse treatment. NIDA Research Monographs 119:150–154.

Mello NK, Mendelson JH. 1992. Primate studies of the behavioral pharmacology of buprenorphine. NIDA Research Monographs 121:61–100.

Mello NK, Mendelson JH, Bree MP. 1981. Naltrexone effects on morphine and food self-administration in morphine-dependent rhesus monkeys. Journal of Pharmacology and Experimental Therapeutics 218:550–557.

Meng F, Xie GX, Thompson RC, Mansour A, Goldstein A, Watson SJ, Akil H. 1993. Cloning and pharmacological characterization of a rat kappa-opioid receptor. Proceedings of the National Academy of Sciences (USA) 90:9954–9958.

Metzger DS, Cornish J, Woody GE, McLellan AT, Druley P, O'Brien CP. 1989. Naltrexone in federal probationers. NIDA Research Monograph 95:465–466.

Moratalla R, Vickers EA, Robertson HA, Cochran BH, Graybiel AM. 1993. Coordinate expression of c-fos and jun B is induced in the rat striatum by cocaine. Journal of Neuroscience 13:423–433.

Nestler EJ. 1992. Molecular mechanisms of drug addiction. Journal of Neuroscience 12:2439–2450.

Nestler EJ, Greengard P. 1994. Protein phosphorylation and the regulation of neuronal function. In: Siegel GJ, ed. Basic Neurochemistry: Molecular, Cellular, and Medical Aspects. 5th ed. New York: Raven Press. 449–474.

Nestler EJ, Hope BT, Widnell KL. 1993. Drug addiction: a model for the molecular basis of neural plasticity. Neuron 11:995–1006.

North RA. 1979. Opiates, opioid peptides and single neurons. Life Sciences 24:1527–1546.

O'Brien CP. 1975. Experimental analysis of conditioning factors in human narcotic addiction. Pharmacological Reviews 27:535–543.

O'Brien CP, Childress AR, McLellan AT, Ehrman R. 1992. Classical conditioning in drug dependent humans. Annals of the New York Academy of Sciences 654:400–415.

Pratt JA, ed. 1991. The Biological Bases of Drug Tolerance and Dependence. London: Academic Press.

Preston KL, Bigelow GE. 1991. Subjective and discriminative effects of drugs. Behavioral Pharmacology 2:293–313.

Robbins SJ, Ehrman RN, Childress AR, O'Brien CP. 1992. Using cue reactivity to screen medications for cocaine abuse: a test of amantadine hydrochloride. Addictive Behaviors 17:491–499.

Robertson MW, Leslie CA, Bennett JP. 1991. Apparent synaptic dopamine deficiency induced by withdrawal from chronic cocaine treatment. Brain Research 538:337–339.

Rose JE, Levin ED. 1992. Concurrent agonist-antagonist administration for the analysis and treatment of drug dependence. Pharmacology, Biochemistry and Behavior 41:219–226.

Rounsaville BJ, Weissman MM, Wilber C, Kleber HD. 1982. The heterogeneity of psychiatric disorders in treated opiate addicts. Archives of General Psychiatry 39:161–168.

Satel SL, Price LH, Palumbo JM, McDougle CJ, Krystal JH, Gawin F, Charney DS, Heninger GR, Kleber HD. 1991. Clinical phenomenology and neurobiology of cocaine abstinence: a prospective inpatient study. American Journal of Psychiatry 148:1712–1716.

Simon EJ, Hiller JM. 1994. Opioid peptides and opioid receptors. In: Siegel GJ, ed. Basic Neurochemistry: Molecular, Cellular and Medical Aspects, 5th ed. New York: Raven Press. 321–339.

Spealman RD. 1992. Use of cocaine-discrimination techniques for preclinical evaluation of candidate therapeutics for cocaine dependence. NIDA Research Monographs 119:175–179.

Spealman RD, Bergman J, Madras BK, Kamien JB, Melia KF. 1992. Role of D1 and D2 dopamine receptors in the behavioral effects of cocaine. Neurochemistry International 20:147S–152S.

Terenius L, O'Brien CP. 1991. Receptors and endogenous ligands: implications for addiction. In: O'Brien CP, Jaffe JH, eds. Addictive States. New York: Raven Press. 123–130.

Vocci F. 1993. Memorandum to the IOM Committee on Medication Development and Research at NIDA re: MDD's chemical synthesis program and biochemical and animal behavior screening programs. December 5, 1993.

Volkow N, Fowler JS, Wolf AP, Schlyer D, Shiue CY, Alpert R, Dewey SL, Logan J, Bendriem B, Christman D. 1990. Effects of chronic cocaine abuse on postsynaptic dopamine receptors. American Journal of Psychiatry 147:719–724.

Wang JB, Imai Y, Eppler CM, Gregor P, Spivak CE, Uhl GR. 1993. Mu opiate receptor: CDNA cloning and expression. Proceedings of the National Academy of Sciences (USA) 90:10230–10234.

Weddington WW, Brown BS, Haertzen CA, Cone EJ, Dax EM, Herning RI, Michaelson BS. 1990. Changes in mood, craving, and sleep during short-term abstinence reported by male cocaine addicts. Archives of General Psychiatry 47:861–868.

Weiss F, Markou A, Lorang MT, Koob GF. 1992. Basal extracellular dopamine levels in the nucleus accumbens are decreased during cocaine withdrawal after unlimited-access self-administration. Brain Research 593:314–318.

WHO (World Health Organization). 1990. Draft of chapter V: mental and behavioural disorders. Clinical descriptions and diagnostic guidelines. International Classification of Diseases, 10th rev. Geneva: WHO. As cited in: Jaffe JH. 1992. Current concepts of addiction. In: O'Brien CP, Jaffe JH, eds. Addictive States. New York: Raven Press.

Wikler A. 1973. Dynamics of drug dependence: implications of a conditioning theory for research and treatment. Archives of General Psychiatry 28:611–616.

Wise RA, Hoffman DC. 1992. Localization of drug reward mechanisms by intracranial injections. Synapse 10:247–263.

Woods JH, Bertalmio AJ, Young AM, Essman WD, Winger G. 1988. Receptor mechanisms of opioid drug discrimination. In: Colpaert FC, Balster RL, eds. Transduction Mechanisms of Drug Stimuli. Berlin: Springer-Verlag. 95–106.

Woods JH, France CP, Winger G, Bertalmio AJ, Schwarz-Stevens K. 1993. Opioid abuse liability assessment in rhesus monkeys. In: Akil H, Herz A, Simon EJ, eds. Handbook of Experimental Pharmacology. Vol. 104, Opioids I. Berlin: Springer-Verlag. 609–632.

Woolverton WL, Kleven MS. 1992. Assessment of new medications for stimulant abuse treatment. NIDA Research Monographs 119:155–159.

Yasuda K, Raynor K, Kong H, Breder CD, Takeda J, Reisine T, Bell GI. 1993. Cloning and functional comparison of kappa and delta opioid receptors from mouse brain. Proceedings of the National Academy of Sciences (USA) 90:6736–6740.

Young AM, Herling S. 1986. Drugs as reinforcers: studies in laboratory animals. In: Goldberg SR, Stolerman IP, eds. Behavioral Analysis of Drug Dependence. Orlando: Academic Press. 9–67.

Young ST, Porrino LJ, Iadarola MJ. 1991. Cocaine induces striatal c-fos-immunoreactive proteins via dopaminergic D_1 receptors. Proceedings of the National Academy of Sciences (USA) 88:1291–1295.

3

Assessment of the
Medications Development Division

This chapter describes and assesses the activities of the National Institute on Drug Abuse (NIDA) Medications Development Division (MDD), which was established in 1990 to bring new medications for the treatment of drug addiction to market. This assessment is based on written materials supplied by MDD and meetings between the Institute of Medicine committee and representatives of MDD, the Food and Drug Administration (FDA), the Drug Enforcement Administration (DEA), and the pharmaceutical industry. In addition, over 20 persons knowledgeable about MDD were interviewed at length by an outside consultant. (List of acknowledgements in Appendix A).

STRUCTURE AND FUNCTIONS OF THE
MEDICATIONS DEVELOPMENT DIVISION

Mission and History

In recognition of the need to stimulate the availability of medications to treat drug addiction, the Anti-Drug Abuse Act of 1988 (Public Law 100-690) authorized funds for a drug discovery and development program within NIDA. Beginning with an appropriation of $8 million in 1988, NIDA launched a Medications Development Program in its Division of Preclinical Research. Building on this program, NIDA formally established the Medications Development Division in 1990. The ADAMHA Reorganization Act (Public Law 102-321), enacted in July 1992, moved NIDA from the Alcohol, Drug Abuse, and

74

Mental Health Administration (ADAMHA) to the National Institutes of Health (NIH). The act authorized a Medications Development Program at $85 million in fiscal year (FY) 1993 and $95 million in FY 1994, although actual funding has been only about one-third of the authorization.

The primary strategy adopted by MDD is to work with industry to perform the research and development necessary to secure FDA marketing approval for new medications to treat drug addiction. A more complete description of MDD, including the mission of each of its five branches, is in Appendix B.

The division, with a FY 1993 budget of about $36 million and a staff of 33, appears to have the capacity to fund the development of at best only a small number of drugs to the point of marketability for treating drug addiction (Chapter 7 for costs of drug development). MDD does not operate inhouse laboratories or clinical-development programs to fulfill its mission. Rather, it manages this work through multiple external instruments, such as contracts, grants, and interagency and collaborative agreements. For example, MDD has an interagency agreement with the Department of Veterans Affairs (DVA) and pays it to conduct large, multicenter clinical trials on promising treatment agents. In this fashion, MDD could, in principle, develop a drug from the point of discovery through FDA approval and then license it for marketing and distribution (and perhaps manufacturing) by a commercial partner.

Although MDD might in theory develop a drug on its own in that fashion, it is structured and funded instead to leverage its resources by seeking private partners and offering them incentives to collaborate in the development of medications for the treatment of drug addiction. The incentives offered by the division include

- The assumption of some—if not all—of the costs of clinical development by performing the clinical studies for the private partner.
- The provision of technical assistance (e.g., screening chemicals for utility as anti-addiction medications and designing and analyzing the results of clinical trials).
- The provision of assistance in working with FDA to secure marketing approval.

MDD's role as a catalyst of a private sponsor's activity can be very versatile. It might in one instance be limited to in vitro screening of a sponsor's drug or in another might be as extensive as carrying out nearly all the development activities, including the fulfillment of regulatory requirements of FDA and DEA.

Research Focus on Opiates and Cocaine

MDD's research is concerned almost exclusively with identifying and developing treatment for opiate and cocaine addiction. The focus on opiate research is an outgrowth of NIDA's historical strength in this research. MDD's more recent focus on cocaine treatment, however, stemmed from criticism of NIDA's alleged neglect of cocaine and crack addiction (GAO, 1990). The criticism prompted the division—at its very inception—to concentrate its resources on developing a portfolio of medications for both opiate and cocaine addiction. Ironically, the almost exclusive focus on those two kinds of addiction has engendered criticism from some quarters that MDD is neglecting other kinds, such as alcoholism and nicotine addiction. However, the division maintains that its focus on opiate and cocaine treatments is justified for three reasons (C. Grudzinskas, NIDA, personal communication):

• Opiate- and cocaine-dependent individuals are disproportionately responsible for violent crimes and for the transmission of the human immunodeficiency virus (HIV).
• The private sector has failed to provide an adequate number of treatments for opiate addiction and has provided no treatments for cocaine addiction, although it is actively pursuing treatments for nicotine addiction and already has products on the market.
• Alcoholism research is the purview of another NIH institute, the National Institute on Alcohol Abuse and Alcoholism (NIAAA).

For the purposes of this report, the Institute of Medicine (IOM) committee accepts this justification and current emphasis of MDD on opiate and cocaine addictions; although the committee recognizes that the two addictive drugs that are most important with respect to morbidity, mortality, and economic costs are alcohol and nicotine.

Program Objectives

MDD's mission statement describes its program objective: the development of new medications to treat drug addiction. Furthermore, MDD has articulated specific program objectives in its 1992 document *Five Year Strategic Plan* (NIDA, 1992). These can be simply stated:

- To screen at least 200 chemicals each year for possible therapeutic value.
- To develop three new opiate medications in the next 5 years.
- To develop one or two new cocaine medications in the next 5 years.

Organizational Structure

MDD is one of five research divisions of NIDA. It is organized like a small pharmaceutical company with five branches (Chemistry/Pharmaceutics, Pharmacology/Toxicology, Clinical Trials, Biometrics, and Regulatory Affairs) that cover the usual drug-development activities from preclinical research to regulation (see Appendix B for division and branch mission statements). As is typical in the industry, the division's programs are carried out in a matrix management style by teams drawn from the branches. There are four programs:

- Opiate Treatment Discovery Program.
- Opiate Treatment Clinical Program.
- Cocaine Treatment Discovery Program.
- Cocaine Treatment Clinical Program.

As an example, the Cocaine Treatment Discovery Program attempts to acquire at least 200 chemicals each year from the pharmaceutical industry and other sources. On acquisition, each chemical is subjected to a battery of in vitro biochemical assays and in vivo pharmacological and behavioral studies to identify promising therapeutic agents to treat cocaine addiction. To carry out all the steps necessary, the program draws staff from each of MDD's five branches who have the appropriate expertise.

All of MDD's outside research and development is managed by three of the five branches—the Chemistry/Pharmaceutics Branch, the Pharmacology/Toxicology Branch, and the Clinical Trials Branch. The other two branches provide technical support for those three. The Regulatory Affairs Branch seeks industry partners, negotiates Cooperative Research and Development Agreements (CRADAs), secures the regulatory approvals necessary to conduct research, and serves as a critical link to many other private and public programs. The Biometrics Branch, a staff of statisticians, provides assistance in protocol design, data management, and statistical analysis.

Budget Process

In a departure from most NIH institutes, the overall budget for NIDA (in addition to that for NIAAA and the National Institute of Mental Health) is currently submitted to Congress by the President in what is called a "bypass budget." This budget undergoes the same appropriations process once it is delivered to Congress, but it is developed and presented to the Office of Management and Budget without being reviewed by NIDA's parent agency, the Department of Health and Human Services (DHHS). The submission of a bypass budget was authorized only for 2 years (FY 1993 and FY 1994) by the ADAMHA Reorganization Act of 1992 in an effort to ensure continuity of funding for NIDA and to avoid competition with already-established NIH institutes.

Neither the budget request nor the Congressional appropriation for NIDA is specifically allocated down to the level of each NIDA division. Rather, the budget is broken into major categories covering all the divisions, such as research grants, centers, training, and contracts (Table 3.1). Once funds are appropriated to NIDA within these categories, the divisions must compete against each other for funding. The competition must take into account that most of each division's budget is already committed to continuing prior grants and contracts.

Resources and Funding Instruments

Despite MDD's authorization of $95 million in FY 1994, the actual appropriations have been far less, although they have been increasing. MDD's budget has grown steadily since 1988 (when it was known as the Medications Development Program), climbing from $8 million in FY 1988 to $40 million in FY 1994. Similarly, the number of full-time equivalent personnel (FTEs) has increased from 10 in FY 1990 to 33 in FY 1994.

MDD has no internal laboratory or clinical research capabilities, so virtually all its budget is spent on grants, contracts, and interagency agreements aimed at drug development. In general, about half the MDD budget is devoted to grants and the other half to contracts (which include interagency agreements). The balance between grants and contracts has shifted because in the early years of the division most of the funds were dispersed through contracts. The majority of the budget (about 60–65 percent) was spent on contracts in FY 1990–1992. However, in FY 1993, contracts consumed about half, or $18.5 million, of the total budget of $35.6 million.

MDD is not the only division in NIDA that is involved in medication development. Some activities in other NIDA divisions support medication development, and these, with the MDD functions, are linked into an overall program, the Medications Development Program. The other NIDA divisions that contribute to the Medications Development Program are the Division of Basic Research, the Division of Clinical Research, the Division of Epidemiology and Prevention Research, and the Addiction Research Center (NIDA's intramural research facility). In terms of funding, however, the MDD budget constitutes approximately 80 percent of the Medications Development Program.

TABLE 3.1 NIDA FY 1995 Budget Appropriation

	Number	Amount
Research Grants		
Research projects	828	266,728,000
Research centers	33	46,146,000
Other research	118	18,853,000
Training		
Individual awards	77	1,640,000
Institutional awards	277	7,668,000
Research and development contracts	64	41,330,000
FTEs		
Intramural research	107	24,747,000
Research management and support	279	30,580,000
Total	386	437,692,000
Clinical Trials		(79,200,000)

SOURCE: U.S. DHHS, 1993.

Types of Grants and Contracts

There are many different types of NIH grants and contracts. The two types of grants used most by MDD are R01 (investigator-initiated grants) and R18 (research-demonstration grants). The R18 category is also called a treatment-research unit (TRU). These units can be likened to a type of center grant,[1] and they range in size from $1.5 to $2 million each. Under a TRU, funds may be spent on staff, facilities, and a variety of individual research projects for clinical

---

[1]TRUs are categorized formally as a type of demonstration project. In FY 1995, TRUs will be discontinued and replaced by a formal center grant.

drug treatments. In FY 1993, four TRUs were funded by MDD at a total cost of $9.5 million. TRUs are now being converted to center grants and apply competitively for these grants as they come up for renewal.

Two general types of contracts are used by MDD: the N01 is a typical R&D contract, and the other type is an interagency agreement. In FY 1993, about half the total contract budget of $18.5 million was spent on R&D contracts and the other half on interagency agreements.

Interagency Agreements

Through interagency agreements with the DVA Cooperative Studies Program, MDD has gained the capacity to undertake large-scale Phase III clinical trials. Indeed, an overall capacity to carry out two large-scale clinical trials at the same time is now available and operationally tested. As part of the recent development of levo-alpha-acetylmethadol (LAAM), DVA (supported by MDD) conducted a 25-site trial involving 625 participants. Simultaneously, a 12-site, 735-patient trial of buprenorphine was also undertaken.

Under this interagency agreement, MDD has spent about $6 million to purchase access to DVA resources, such as physicians, statisticians, clinical coordinators, computer operators, and all other types of professionals and facilities needed for clinical trials and the analysis of their results. DVA has the ability to coordinate and analyze data from both DVA and non-DVA sites. This coordinating function is performed by DVA's Cooperative Studies Program in Perry Point, Maryland. Trials at DVA sites are usually far less expensive than those at other hospitals or clinics because overhead and physicians' salaries are covered by DVA and the administrative costs are lower than those of a study organized and monitored by a contract research organization. The clinical trial for LAAM cost $6,000 per patient per year—a cost estimated by MDD to be about half that for a trial performed by a commercial contractor (F. Vocci, NIDA, personal communication).

Other interagency agreements with DVA cover Phase I-II clinical studies in individual DVA hospitals in Los Angeles, Philadelphia, and Washington, D.C.

To address preclinical and toxicological research and development needs, MDD has several other interagency agreements with other NIH institutes, the Environmental Protection Agency, and the Armed Forces Institute of Pathology.

CRADAs

MDD's preferred means of collaborating with industry in the development of drugs is through CRADAs, contracts governing collaborative research and development. A CRADA is not a funding instrument for academic investigators or private companies, but an agreement between government and industry to work collaboratively to spur commercialization of a product. It contains a research plan, including a protocol, and describes what each party contributes. The government is permitted to provide access to researchers, facilities, and in-kind services but is not permitted to contribute funds (although it may receive them from the industry partner). A CRADA also defines in advance who will receive intellectual property rights, and it gives the industry partner the right to negotiate for exclusive licensing of any patent that the government obtains during the course of the CRADA, including licensing for a new use of the sponsor's product. For example, the commercial sponsor might obtain exclusive marketing of a new psychoactive compound for the treatment of depression, as well as for drug addiction.

Thus far, MDD has succeeded in negotiating two CRADAs with industry partners, both for potential treatments for cocaine addiction: one for Phase II clinical research on gepirone with Bristol Myers Squibb, and the other for Phase II research for bupropion with Burroughs Wellcome. MDD is in the process of developing other CRADAs, including one with Reckitt & Colman Pharmaceutic-als, Inc., for preclinical and clinical research on buprenorphine alone or in combination with naloxone for the treatment of opiate addiction (NIH, 1993).

In addition to defining intellectual property rights clearly in advance, the reason that a CRADA is useful to both MDD and a private partner is that it is much more flexible than a contract. Contracts take a long time to award and are difficult to alter once they are in place. But a CRADA can be started relatively quickly (under a letter of intent) and is resilient enough to accommodate changes, such as those often requested by FDA in the course of its evaluation of human trials.

MDD officials reported to the committee that, although they are quite willing to use CRADAs as a mechanism for collaborating with pharmaceutical companies in conducting clinical studies, many potential partners are uninterested in CRADAs because of a controversial provision that goes well beyond MDD—the reasonable-pricing clause. This clause is a relatively recent policy requirement in all CRADAs negotiated by DHHS, and is currently being re-examined by NIH. The manner in which the reasonable-pricing clause acts as a disincentive to the private sector is presented in Chapter 9 with a committee recommendation.

Screening Agreements

A screening agreement is the vehicle that MDD uses to obtain chemicals for testing from industry, academe, etc. These agreements are similar to the more commonly known material-transfer agreements. Screening agreements spell out the terms of MDD's acquisition of chemicals to carry out in vitro assays and in vivo pharmacological testing. The purpose of the assays is to evaluate which of the many compounds already synthesized by drug firms hold potential for further development for human use. All the testing performed by MDD under screening agreements is carried out through contracts, and there is no charge to the sponsors. Under a screening agreement, a commercial sponsor provides confidential information about the chemical structure, physical properties, and biological activity of its compound. The results of MDD's screening tests are given to the sponsor and are entered into NIDA's structure-activity database. Prior to 1994 the information from NIDA's screening tests remained confidential for only 3 years. That agreement had hindered MDD's ability to acquire compounds and affected MDD's capability to develop its screening program adequately because many companies did not want their confidential data to be made public. Thus, in 1994 MDD revised their original screening agreement and now all screening data from industry compounds will remain confidential. That change in policy should have a beneficial effect on MDD's screening program. The company benefits from the screening agreement by retaining all pre-existing rights to its chemicals because the standard screening agreement stipulates that the testing does not constitute "invention" under the patent laws.

Training

Increasing support for the training of researchers and clinician investigators in drug-abuse research and treatment has been recognized by NIDA officials as a particularly important goal. The General Accounting Office has also cited research training as a field in which it thinks that NIDA should expand its efforts (GAO, 1990).

Specifically with respect to medication development, two major factors appear to be limiting the training of scientists and clinical investigators in this field. The first is the scarcity of training funds. In the FY 1994 bypass-budget request, NIDA asked to raise the number of trainees from 297 to 440 full-time training positions. However, only modest increases were funded.

The second factor is a lack of interest of young physicians in drug-abuse research and treatment. This is a general professional problem related to the relative isolation of treatment of drug abuse from the mainstream of academic medicine and medical practice, the personal health risks of working with patients who often have such other serious illnesses as HIV infection or tuberculosis, the difficulties of conducting high-quality clinical research in the social environment in which the bulk of addiction occurs, the perceived low respectability of the field, and the involvement of many patients with crime or the criminal justice system. Those are difficult obstacles to overcome, but the committee believes that the designation of several major national drug abuse research centers (Chapter 2 and 6) will help to attract scientists and physicians.

MDD has proposed a different approach to help to rectify the scarcity of physicians who have training in drug-addiction research: creating a $500,000–1,000,000 training program in FY 1994 (C. Grudzinskas, NIDA, personal communication). This program would be administered through FDA's Staff College and would provide stipends for 9–12 clinicians to receive 3 years of training through rotations at three federal programs: MDD, the FDA Pilot Drug Evaluation staff, and the NIDA Addiction Research Center.

Another incentive to attract clinicians to the drug-addiction field that NIDA would like to be able to offer is a loan-repayment program. There is a precedent for this type of incentive: under new legislative authority, the National Institute of Allergy and Infectious Diseases is able to help its employees to repay educational loans in exchange for service in acquired immune deficiency syndrome (AIDS) research. The desired authority for clinicians in drug treatment and research would be along the lines of this model.

The lack of trained clinicians in the field of drug addiction is viewed as an obstacle to progress, not only by MDD in realizing its goals of medication development, but also in treatment and clinical research. Chapter 6 discusses training issues in greater depth.

RELATIONSHIPS WITH OTHER FEDERAL AGENCIES AND THE PRIVATE SECTOR

Food and Drug Administration

MDD and FDA are parts of the same agency, the Public Health Service (PHS), and are also linked through FDA's drug review process. NIDA may also sponsor investigational new drug (IND) applications.[2] To receive an IND, NIDA or any other sponsor has to submit an extensive application to FDA containing the results of laboratory and animal testing, details of manufacturing processes, and clinical-research plans. The granting of an IND gives the authority to begin testing in humans. NIDA or its industry partner is also responsible for meeting all FDA requirements to conduct clinical trials and obtain evidence necessary to win marketing approval. Chapter 7 further examines the role of FDA and its influence on the private sector in developing anti-addiction medications.

As part of the process of developing LAAM, MDD has reached an excellent working relationship with the FDA Pilot Drug Evaluation group. This relation-

---

[2]NIDA holds INDs for LAAM, buprenorphine, and depot naltrexone.

ship includes continuing communication, discussion of problems as they arise, and trust between the staffs of the two organizations. FDA has also developed special software to allow sponsors to submit clinical data on-line electronically as they are entered into the sponsor's database; this approach played a crucial role in the rapid approval of LAAM.

FDA and NIDA also participate in the process for scheduling drugs of abuse and in the promulgation of regulations on treatment standards for the use of narcotics in treating drug addiction. Under the Comprehensive Drug Abuse Prevention and Control Act of 1970, the secretary of DHHS must issue regulations that describe how any new narcotic medication can be administered and used in narcotic treatment programs. Regulations under this law related to the use of methadone in treating opiate addiction have been in place since 1972 and were amended to accommodate the recent approval of LAAM (FDA, 1993). Those regulations are further discussed in Chapter 8 and are considered in detail in a forthcoming IOM report on methadone regulations (IOM, 1995).

Drug Enforcement Administration

Under the Controlled Substances Act, DEA and NIDA have defined roles in the scheduling of drugs of abuse.[3] Scheduling is a means of restricting the availability of drugs to ensure that they are accessible for medical purposes but not for illicit trafficking. The law requires that NIDA's parent agency, DHHS, evaluate the medical utility and the abuse potential of a narcotic drug and recommend in which of five schedules—or categories—a drug should be placed. DHHS relies heavily on NIDA and FDA for preparing this evaluation. Once DHHS submits its evaluation and recommendation to DEA, DEA is legally bound by the Controlled Substances Act to place a drug in a schedule that is not more restrictive than that recommended by DHHS (Chapter 7).

In addition to their roles with respect to drug scheduling, NIDA and DEA are brought together under additional requirements of the Controlled Substances Act. If NIDA (or a private sponsor) holds an IND to test a Schedule I drug (i.e., a drug with no accepted medical use and a high potential for abuse), the sponsor is required to have its research sites registered with DEA. DEA must inspect each research site and grant a permit before a Schedule I substance may be shipped to that site. This requirement for individual inspections led to lengthy delays in NIDA's Phase III study of LAAM and is a disincentive to industry in

---

[3]By statute, the formal relationship is between DEA and the secretary of DHHS. The secretary has delegated this authority to the assistant secretary for health as the director of PHS. In practice, most of the negotiations between DEA and PHS are conducted by representatives of DEA and the two PHS agencies, FDA and NIDA.

the development of anti-addiction medications. Additionally, there are state controlled substances acts that have an effect on pharmaceutical R&D (Chapter 8).

Office of Protection from Research Risks

NIH's Office of Protection from Research Risks (OPRR) reviews and archives all consent and approval forms for NIH-sponsored research. For any U.S. human trials, participants must give informed consent, and the protocol and consent form must be approved by an institutional review board (IRB), a special review body set up by each institution that sponsors research. These are basic requirements of ethical clinical research and of the federal regulations for the protection of human subjects. In arranging for the recent LAAM study, obtaining IRB approval of individual study sites became unusually complex, primarily because LAAM was, until it was approved by FDA, a Schedule I substance under the Controlled Substances Act. It is useful to note these complexities in some detail because they illustrate the procedural problems that make clinical research on anti-addiction compounds difficult; they will complicate future clinical trials involving narcotics unless new policy solutions can be found.

In the LAAM study, the numerous sites conducting the trials were not traditional research institutions; rather, they were methadone clinics, many of which did not have pre-existing IRBs to evaluate protocols and consent forms. Furthermore, these clinics did not have on file with OPRR an assurance[4] that they would comply with all human-subjects regulations or the required registration. To solve that problem, MDD helped each methadone clinic either to establish its own IRB or to use an existing IRB in another institution that had the competence to evaluate drug-addiction research. MDD, through DVA, also helped each methadone clinic to file with OPRR a single-project assurance containing a statement that all human-subjects protections would be complied with during the study, a list of IRB members, and a proposed informed-consent form. If NIDA supports future studies at the same clinics, a new single project assurance will need to be filed for each clinic.

The history of consent forms and protocol reviews in the LAAM study illustrates the kinds of issues that bring procedural complexity to multicenter trials (Vocci, 1993, presentation to IOM committee). The consent form became the mechanism in this trial for informing study participants that, in spite of a general policy in clinical trials that personal information is confidential, this policy would be broken in the LAAM study if a patient were found to have a reportable transmissible disease (e.g., tuberculosis) or made voluntary disclosures

---

[4]Most institutions file a multiproject assurance with OPRR to cover many projects at once for a period of 5 years.

about committing child abuse. To develop a consensus on these points, MDD developed additional language for the consent form to provide greater detail about the limits of confidentiality. The consent form had to be agreed on by the appropriate IRBs, the DVA Human Subjects Protection Committee (because some of the sites were located in the DVA medical system), FDA, and OPRR. MDD also helped research sites to obtain confidentiality certificates to protect patients' privacy (in the event of a court challenge) and to protect research confidentiality.

All those activities, although time-consuming and labor-intensive, would have been conducted by the sponsor of any large, multicenter clinical trial, regardless of the type of compound being tested, as part of compliance with FDA and DHHS regulations. Because LAAM was a Schedule I substance, however, an additional set of procedural requirements driven by the Controlled Substances Act came into play: multiple reviews of the protocol to ensure that it met the scientific requirements of FDA; the DEA regulations related to recordkeeping, security, and diversion; the methadone regulation of DHHS; and the counterpart narcotic regulations of each state that contained a participating clinic. The MDD staff estimates that about 15 drafts of the protocol, with iterative consultation and agreement, were necessary. Nevertheless, one state (California) could never agree, because one point in its drug regulations is more stringent than the federal methadone regulations, so no clinic in California participated in the study (F. Vocci, NIDA, personal communication). The committee realizes that individual state regulations may negatively impact the ability to conduct clinical trials. See Chapter 8 for further discussion of state regulations.

Pharmaceutical Industry

The pharmaceutical industry plays an integral role in the drug-development strategy adopted by MDD. As stated earlier, MDD offers drug firms both resources and technical assistance to bring a medication to market. MDD prefers a very active industry role, but at the very least a partner is needed to market and distribute any medication that is jointly developed.

Another key role for industry is to provide MDD with chemicals to screen for potential therapeutic value. MDD or the industry partner may proceed with development if a compound shows therapeutic promise after a battery of screening tests. The role of screening in drug discovery is discussed in Chapter 2.

In addition to working with individual companies, MDD has received input from the Pharmaceutical Manufacturers Association (PMA, now the Pharmaceutical Research and Manufacturers of America, PhRMA), a trade association whose members are some of the largest U.S. drug manufacturers. In 1990, PMA created the PMA Commission on Medicines for Treatment of Drug Dependence and Abuse (CDDA), and this commission has, through a subcommittee, presented to MDD its perspective on a strategy for screening potential treatments for cocaine addiction. A technical subcommittee of CDDA has provided information about methods for clinical and statistical design that are often used in medication-development clinical trials.

ASSESSMENT OF THE MEDICATIONS DEVELOPMENT DIVISION

MDD has made considerable progress in the 4 years since its inception. The committee's impressions of the specific accomplishments of the division are noted here.

Staff and Resources

The committee recognizes that MDD appears to be hampered by lack of personnel, and it is the understanding of the committee that any large increase of funds could not benefit the program unless accompanied by additional staff. The committee, however, did not evaluate in detail the staff and resources devoted to various activities of MDD. Although the current budget of $40 million and the 33-FTE staff might be adequate to support the development of a small portfolio of products based on drugs that are already in use, the committee believes that they are insufficient to support basic research (Chapter 2).

Furthermore, given the full panoply of responsibilities needed to accomplish the mission of MDD (see mission statements in Appendix B), the staff appears overextended. For example, MDD has only one physician on staff, but a clinical trial can be best designed and monitored by a physician working with the support of other research professionals. Thus, the clinical trials must be designed and monitored by current staff in addition to their numerous other responsibilities. Similarly, the requirements of the screening program appear to need additional qualified staff, especially if NIDA and MDD decide to implement the committee's recommendations for improving the cocaine screening program (Chapter 2). The committee is aware, however, of the budgetary and hiring constraints and suggests ways to overcome them in Chapter 2.

Drug-Discovery Programs

The committee commends MDD for its interest in establishing screening programs for new compounds that might have anti-opiate or anti-cocaine activity and for its screening efforts. As noted in Chapter 2, however, the anti-opiate field is relatively mature with respect to the availability of scientific methods for the discovery of anti-opiate compounds, whereas the anti-cocaine field is in its infancy. Because of the lack of established in vitro screening methods and validated animal models that are predictive in humans for anti-cocaine medications, the committee feels that there is a need for basic research to develop laboratory models of critical behavioral characteristics of the addictive process. In addition, improvement of such methods and models should be given high priority for grant and contract support by MDD (see elaboration and recommendations in Chapter 2).

The committee also supports the limited screening of compounds with the methods already identified by MDD with the advice of the PMA CDDA to gain experience and build effective working relationships with industry partners. However, the committee does not see such screening as the primary route to identifying new treatments for cocaine addiction, nor as essential to progress, at least in the near term. The committee recommends that emphasis be given to the early clinical evaluation of known psychoactive compounds in moderate-sized, controlled clinical trials for the early determination of efficacy. Those compounds might be drugs approved for other uses, drugs under development by pharmaceutical companies, or compounds related to such drugs.

Clinical Trials

The committee commends MDD for completing the development of LAAM and recognizes that MDD analyzed a file of accumulated data on some 6,300 patients and negotiated with FDA a final Phase III clinical trial necessary for LAAM's approval. The committee is impressed that MDD has gained invaluable experience and built an effective clinical-investigator network and administrative base that can be used for the conduct of Phase III studies on other anti-addiction drugs. Inasmuch as the pharmaceutical industry considers the difficulty of organizing and conducting clinical studies to be an obstacle to its interest in this field (Chapter 9), MDD's building of a major, continuing clinical-trial capability represents a resource of permanent value to both MDD and the private sector. The committee encourages MDD to maintain this resource and build on it further in its partnership arrangements with individual drug firms.

With respect to the conduct of clinical research in patients with drug addiction, the committee is impressed that such research is greatly complicated from an administrative point of view and that costs are increased by the presence of multiple independent regulations, including the IND regulations of FDA, the narcotic-treatment regulations of DHHS, the DEA regulations related to recordkeeping, security, and scheduling, and state scheduling and treatment regulations. Those regulations are major disincentives to the private sector in the development of anti-addiction compounds; they are discussed extensively in Chapters 7 and 8, where several recommendations are proposed for overcoming those barriers.

Clinical-Research Training

Patients with drug-abuse problems often require diagnostic assessment and treatment for such sequelae as liver disease, HIV, other infection, and trauma. A large number of patients with primary psychiatric disease also require treatment for drug abuse (Beeder and Millman, 1992). But the number of physicians specially trained to care for this large patient population is small, as are the numbers of sites and clinical investigators for studying drug abuse (Chapter 6). As discussed earlier, the appeal of this field is limited by the stigma of drug addiction, the noncompliance of drug-dependent individuals as subjects in clinical trials, the risk of infectious diseases that afflict these patients, and the general lack of insurance coverage for drug-abuse treatment. The lack of clinical research and treatment centers has and will continue to have an impact on MDD's ability to carry out sophisticated clinical studies of pharmacological and other treatments in those patients.

The committee noted in Chapter 2 that the designation of national drug abuse research centers will attract qualified young physicians into the field of drug abuse. The committee believes that such centers should provide training and drug-abuse education to clinicians as a mechanism of encouraging the development of medical expertise (Chapter 6).

Other incentives that might attract physicians early in their training to pursue careers in the field of drug-abuse research and treatment are awarding of certificates of "added qualification" on completion of at least a year of full-time formal training in this subspecialty, educational-loan forgiveness programs, and reasonably paid fellowship programs that are competitive with private-sector salaries.

Relationships with Regulatory Agencies

MDD has established an excellent working relationship with the Pilot Drug Evaluation staff of FDA, particularly in the last few years as a result of the effective collaboration that brought the development of LAAM to completion. This relationship includes a spirit of trust, reciprocal access (to nonproprietary information), the establishment of a data linkage that permits data from NIDA clinical trials to be transmitted to FDA for early scrutiny and analysis as they are entered into the clinical-trials database, and a common commitment to conducting good clinical studies and reviewing the results rapidly. The relationship is an important long-term asset to both agencies. It can serve as the basis for continuing communication and productive effort in the development of future anti-addiction medications and maintaining the scientific independence of NIDA and the regulatory role of FDA. The committee believes that this relationship should be strongly encouraged to continue. To that end, the committee urges a formalization of the relationship between NIDA and FDA (Chapter 9 for discussion and recommendation).

Unfortunately, DEA's role in regulating research and treatment sites has been an obstacle for MDD. The LAAM clinical trial was delayed by 3–6 months because of the time DEA required to inspect each of the 24 separate research sites before this Schedule I narcotic could be dispensed in a clinical protocol.

Another major obstacle to drug development is the extraordinary degree of regulation surrounding a treatment after it is approved for marketing. The separate regulatory system resulted from the passage of the Narcotic Addict Treatment Act in 1974. This act, which amended the Controlled Substances Act (21 USC 823), placed drug treatment out of the mainstream of medicine through elaborate requirements for practitioners who dispense narcotics for maintenance or detoxification treatment. The federal requirements, which are enforced by FDA and DEA, include annual registration covering the practitioner's qualifications, security arrangements, recordkeeping, and compliance with treatment standards. Additionally, many states have enacted more stringent treatment regulations (Chapters 8).

Interaction with the Private Sector

The committee commends MDD for its initiatives involving the private sector, although MDD has had difficulties in gaining industry partners and industry chemicals for screening. MDD provides incentives to gain industry partners (e.g., technical assistance, working with FDA for drug approval, and absorbing some of the costs of drug development), but they are not considered strong enough to overcome the numerous obstacles to private-sector investment in the field of anti-addiction medications.

The committee believes that there are two possible explanations for industry's apparent lack of interest in volunteering chemicals from its chemical libraries. The first is that industry and MDD have different expectations about the potential value of these libraries as a resource. To some companies, the libraries represent an investment in the future that must be closely protected. Even though the chemicals might have been archived because of seemingly less immediate commercial potential, the companies recognize that this potential could change overnight if new discoveries are made. Furthermore, rather than turning over a chemical to MDD, a company might prefer to license the chemical to another, usually smaller company for further testing.

The second explanation has been industry discontent with the screening agreement developed by MDD to obtain chemicals for testing. Although the screening agreement assures commercial sponsors the intellectual property rights, the unresolved legal issues between NIH and Burroughs Wellcome over patenting of the AIDS treatment zidovudine (AZT) has created a climate of uncertainty and distrust (Felsenthal, 1993). Prior to 1994 some pharmaceutical companies were also uncomfortable with the provision of the screening agreement that gave MDD the right to disclose the results of its screening of an industry chemical within 3 years. However the screening agreement was changed in 1994 to stipulate that there will unlimited confidentialty of screening test data. This change has made NIDA's policy consistent with other federal drug-development programs (Appendix E).

SUMMARY

MDD has made substantial progress since its inception in 1990. Among its accomplishments are the following:

• It has completed the evaluation of LAAM, a long-acting substitute for methadone for the treatment of opiate addiction, and obtained approval for marketing from FDA.
• It has evaluated several other drugs in major clinical studies, including buprenorphine for opiate addiction, and has sponsored smaller exploratory studies on a variety of compounds.
• It has established through its contractors, especially DVA, a network of experienced clinical investigators.
• It has established an excellent working relationship with FDA.
• To promote drug discovery, it has established a screening program with the goal of identifying new compounds with potential activity against cocaine addiction.
• It has conducted a program of outreach to pharmaceutical companies and worked with the PMA Commission on Medicines for the Treatment of Drug Dependence and Abuse to interest companies in

supplying drugs for screening and in collaborating in the clinical evaluation of their drugs.

Those are major accomplishments for a young organization and provide an excellent base for continuing productivity. However, MDD has had difficulty in stimulating private-sector interest, in acquiring industry partners, and in obtaining a suitable number of compounds for screening. Those difficulties may result from government policy issues that go beyond the power of MDD or NIDA to resolve alone. Nevertheless, it is the opinion of the committee that NIDA can address some of those issues in the context of its current operations: it can increase emphasis on leadership of a public-private cooperative effort, increase emphasis on the early evaluation of promising compounds in clinical pharmacology and early Phase II studies, and create an investigator network that is available to the private sector for Phase III studies. All those moves are aimed at improving NIDA's and MDD's leadership role, management, and strategies for screening. In addition, NIDA can be influential by contributing to the resolution of several current policy issues, including the reasonable-pricing clause in CRADAs, and the difficulty of conducting clinical research under multiple, independent FDA, DEA, DHHS, and state regulations. Those issues are discussed in detail in Chapters 7, 8, and 9 which propose recommendations and options.

CONCLUSIONS AND RECOMMENDATIONS

The committee has noted the need for strong leadership in promoting pharmacotherapy as an important component of our national strategy for combating drug addiction. Leadership must come from many sources, especially the highest levels of the federal bureaucracy (Chapter 9). An important leadership role belongs uniquely to NIDA and especially to MDD for its implementation. MDD must view itself as the leader in stimulating and accelerating development of anti-addiction medications in the United States. That requires a cooperative national endeavor that includes NIDA, academic scientists, and the private sector to integrate the R&D efforts of identifying and developing new drugs for the treatment of addiction. It is not an easy task, given the lack of scientific progress, the limited resources, and the many disincentives to private involvement in this field. Nevertheless, without such leadership, further progress is likely to be haphazard at best.

The committee views this national leadership role in anti-addiction medication development, as one of the key functions of NIDA. MDD should be viewed as the leader of a goal-oriented program that is part of the culture and mission of NIDA and NIH. Consequently, it should be empowered to lead, as well as to fulfill, a scientific and technical mission.

> The committee recommends that NIDA and MDD, in determining how to improve MDD's relationship with industry, evaluate the applicability of the techniques already in use by the Developmental Therapeutics Program of the National Cancer Institute, the National Cooperative Drug Discovery Groups on Acquired Immune Deficiency Syndrome (NCDDG-AIDS) of the National Institute of Allergy and Infectious Disease, and the Anticonvulsant Drug Development Program of the National Institute of Neurological Disorders and Stroke.

Those are all programs (Appendix E) of similar mission within NIH that have established effective working relationships among leading academic and government scientists, FDA, and individual drug companies through a combination of scientific communication, mutual technical assistance, cooperative agreements, and licenses. The intent has been to stimulate success of the enterprise from a national point of view by promoting scientific and technical collaboration and then licensing successful drugs to the private sector for marketing.

With the establishment of MDD, the nation now has a focal point for leadership in the development of therapeutic agents for addiction. In the committee's view, the primary policy responsibility of MDD should be to provide such leadership as a complement to its scientific responsibilities.

Yet, NIDA has been prevented from forming effective partnerships with industry because of the many obstacles and disincentives faced by pharmaceutical companies in the development of anti-addiction medications. Unfortunately, there is little formal literature on drug development specifically as it applies to anti-addiction medications, so the documentation for the information presented, is, in part, testimony from senior executives of the pharmaceutical industry, the committee's expertise, results of a survey of the pharmaceutical, generic-drug, and biotechnology companies (Appendix D); and the June 13, 1994 IOM Workshop (Appendix F). Three major issues were identified as obstacles and disincentives to private sector investment in this field, they include:

- an inadequate science base on addiction and the prevention of relapse, especially for cocaine (Chapter 2);
- an uncertain market environment, including the treatment setting (Chapter 4); treatment financing (Chapter 5); lack of trained specialists for drug addiction treatment and research (Chapter 6); federal and state laws and regulations (Chapters 7 and 8); and market size; pricing issues, societal stigma, liability issues, and difficulties in conducting clinical research (Chapter 9); and
- a lack of sustained federal leadership (Chapter 9).

The committee believes that innovative pharmacotherapies are most likely to be developed through an effective public-private sector partnership with NIDA and a limited number of committed pharmaceutical or biotechnology companies. The remainder of this report identifies the obstacles and disincentives to private sector R&D of anti-addiction medications and offers policy and legislative solutions to overcome the obstacles and stimulate private sector involvement.

REFERENCES

Beeder AB, Millman RB. 1992. Treatment of patients with psychopathology and substance abuse. In: Lowinson JH, Ruiz P, Millman RB, eds. Substance Abuse: A Comprehensive Textbook. 2nd ed. Baltimore: Williams & Wilkins. 675–690.

Felsenthal E. 1993. Who invented AZT? Big bucks are riding on what sleuths find. Wall Street Journal October 21, 1993.

FDA (Food and Drug Administration). 1993. Levo-alpha-acetyl-methadol (LAAM) in maintenance: revision of conditions for use in the treatment of narcotic addiction. July 20, 1993. Federal Register 58(137):38704–38711.

GAO (General Accounting Office). 1990. Drug Abuse: Research on Treatment May Not Address Current Needs. Washington, DC: GAO. GAO HRD-90-114.

IOM (Institute of Medicine). 1995. Federal Regulation of Methadone Treatment. Rettig R, Yarmolinsky A, eds. Washington, DC: National Academy Press.

NIDA (National Institute on Drug Abuse). 1992. National Institute on Drug Abuse Medications Development Program 5 Year Strategic Plan.

NIH (National Institutes of Health). 1993. National Institute on Drug Abuse: announcement of intent to enter a Cooperative Research and Development Agreement (CRADA). May 12, 1993. Federal Register 58(90).

U.S. DHHS (U.S. Department of Health and Human Services). 1993. Justification of Estimates for Appropriations Committees. Fiscal Year 1994. Volume VI, National Institutes of Health.

Vocci FJ, Sorer H. 1992. Pharmacotherapies for treatment of opioid dependence. Journal of Health Care for the Poor and Underserved 3:109–124.

4

Treatment Setting and Effectiveness

This chapter offers a description of the current treatment setting for opiate and cocaine addiction; approaches, patient demographics, and the effectiveness and cost-effectiveness of existing treatments are examined. The treatment system for opiate addiction and that for cocaine addiction are described separately because they offer two distinct markets for pharmaceutical development. For example, a new agonist medication for opiate addiction would most likely compete with the two currently approved pharmacotherapies—methadone and levo-alpha-acetylmethadol (LAAM). Yet, a new medication for cocaine addiction would have little competition, if any, because there is no existing medication that consistently prevents relapse to cocaine addiction.

TREATMENT SETTING

Opiate Addiction

Methadone maintenance with counseling is the treatment of choice for opiate addiction (McLellan et al., 1993). Treatment is provided in tightly regulated programs or clinics, which, until recently have been called "methadone clinics" because methadone has been the only pharmacotherapy approved for opiate addiction. In 1989, the federal treatment regulations were revised and the methadone-specific terms were generalized to say "narcotic treatment" or "narcotic drug" (Federal Register, 1989). Methadone clinics were designated "narcotic treatment programs" to encompass the diversity of available pharmaco-therapies.

Throughout the United States, there are an estimated 650 methadone maintenance programs.[1] They are almost universally located in outpatient facilities, and they must adhere to strict federal and state regulations concerning the use of a narcotic to treat narcotic addiction (Chapters 7 and 8). Since 1987, the number of new clinics nationwide has grown by a modest 16.2 percent (IOM, 1995), despite policies designed to increase access to treatment. In New York, which has the largest opiate-dependent population in the country, only three new methadone clinics have been licensed in 20 years.

A typical methadone maintenance program has four functional areas: a dispensing site, counseling offices, examining rooms, and an administrative area (Ball and Ross, 1991). Patients usually receive a daily oral methadone dose and often have the privilege of a Sunday take-home dose. As the patients progress in treatment, they can be given additional take-home doses, a privilege that is revocable if the patient uses illegal drugs or does not comply with other program requirements. There is wide variation in patient dosing, and many patients receive insufficient doses of methadone (Ball and Ross, 1991; D'Aunno and Vaughn, 1992).

Patients are required to undergo urinalysis to monitor abstinence from illegal drugs while they are in treatment. They also receive counseling at a frequency of usually two individual counseling sessions per month (Ball and Ross, 1991). Patients participate in group counseling and also can receive vocational, rehabilitative, and acquired immune deficiency syndrome (AIDS) counseling. Most clinics are staffed by counselors, nurses, and social workers. Although all clinics are required by federal regulations to have a licensed physician serve as the designated medical director (21 CFR § 291.505), physician time devoted to direct patient care varies greatly depending on the program. Only 16 percent of methadone clinics have full-time physicians on staff (D'Aunno and Vaughn, 1992), and a study of six separate programs noted that physicians treat between 3 percent and 25 percent of patients each week (Ball and Ross, 1991). Physicians and other medical staff members such as nurse practitioners or physician assistants, are responsible for medical management, medications management, physical examinations, and medical education. Nurses are primarily responsible for dispensing medication (Ball and Ross, 1991).

---

[1]This figure is an average of the number of units (574) reported to the National Drug and Alcohol Treatment Unit Survey (NDATUS) in 1992 and the number of dispensing

Utilization of available spaces in methadone clinics is extremely high. In 1992, the nationwide utilization rate was 85.3 percent, according to the 1992 National Drug and Alcoholism Treatment Survey (NDATUS),[2] although other estimates are even higher. The rate is calculated by dividing the actual number of patients by the capacity, or the number of treatment slots. The high rate has led to waiting times for treatment, especially in California and New York, but there are insufficient data on waiting times (IOM, 1995). Some clinics do not keep waiting lists, and some potential patients are so discouraged by waiting lists that they fail to request a slot. A more thorough description of use rates and waiting times is contained in a forthcoming Institute of Medicine report (IOM, 1995).

Most methadone clinics are owned by private, nonprofit organizations, which serve almost 60 percent of patients, according to the 1992 NDATUS. Nonprofit organizations and public agencies together serve more than 75 percent of patients. The private for-profit sector serves about 24 percent of patients, yet it is the fastest growing: from 1987 to 1992, there was a 92.5 percent increase in the number of patients served by privately owned, for-profit facilities. The not-for-profit sector witnessed a patient increase of 18.2 percent. Most of the growth in the for-profit sector has occurred in the southeastern United States, in Texas and California (M. Parrino, American Methadone Treatment Association, personal communication).

Cocaine Addiction

Most cocaine-dependent patients are treated in ambulatory settings (Figure 4.1), but the nature of their care is more diverse. Within ambulatory settings, there are two major modalities of cocaine addiction treatment: out-patient drug-free (ODF) and methadone maintenance. Even though the programs are geared toward opiate addiction, a large percentage of patients in methadone programs also are cocaine users, as described later. A smaller percentage of cocaine-dependent patients are treated in residential settings, in which the two major treatment modalities are therapeutic communities (TCs) and chemical dependency (CD) programs.

---

[2]NDATUS is the most comprehensive survey of all drug abuse and alcoholism treatment facilities throughout the United States. Treatment providers furnish prevalence, use, and financing data to their respective state agencies, which in turn forward the data to the Substance Abuse and Mental Health Services Administration (SAMHSA). Data from the 1992 NDATUS presented in this chapter are not yet published. These data were graciously offered to IOM by Daniel Melnick, Ph.D., acting director, Office of Applied Studies, SAMHSA.

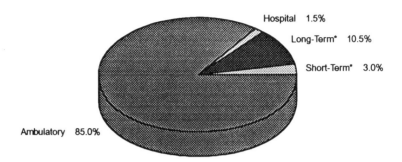

FIGURE 4.1 Percentage of patients in treatment by setting. The population includes patients in treatment for drug dependence and those in treatment for combined dependence on drugs and alcohol. These data are from the National Drug and Alcoholism Treatment Survey, September 30, 1991. *Residential. SOURCE: U.S. DHHS, 1993.

For each of these four treatment modalities for cocaine-dependent patients, Table 4.1 characterizes the setting in which the treatment is administered, the services provided, and the percentage of patients dependent on cocaine prior to treatment.

Outpatient drug-free programs are most common, serving the largest share of patients in treatment (Batten et al., 1993; U.S. DHHS, 1993). The programs provide counseling as the predominant form of treatment, but there is great variation in the array and intensity of counseling services, the quality and training of treatment staff, and the composition of patients. Although about 21 percent of patients in ODF programs are dependent primarily on cocaine or crack, the most commonly abused drugs are alcohol and marijuana (Batten et al., 1992). There also are opiate-dependent patients in treatment; the original goal of ODF programs was to provide a community-based alternative to methadone treatment. ODF programs initially served as "crisis centers" but have evolved into longer term treatment programs (Hubbard et al., 1989). They have increasing allure to patients, insurers, and policy makers because the typical course of treatment is much less expensive than that offered by inpatient and residential programs. Patients are given individual or group psychotherapy or counseling usually once or twice a week, and a treatment episode lasts several months. The term "outpatient drug-free" is somewhat of a misnomer because in many of these programs physicians prescribe medications such as desipramine to treat cocaine craving and clonidine to treat narcotic withdrawal (Anglin and Hser, 1992; C. Wright, FDA, personal communication).

TABLE 4.1 Treatments for Cocaine and Opiate Addiction

Treatment Modality	Setting	Services	Patients Using Cocaine or Opiates in last 30 Days[b]	
			Cocaine[c]	Opiates
Outpatient drug-free	Outpatient	Counseling Prescription drugs[a]	21%	10%
Methadone maintenance	Outpatient	Pharmacotherapy Counseling	39%	83%
Chemical dependency	Residential/ hospital	Counseling Prescription drugs[a]	55%[c] / 42%[d,f]	9%[c] / 14%[d,f]
Therapeutic community	Residential	Counseling	55%[c]	9%[c]

[a]Not all outpatient drug-free programs prescribe medication, but those that do commonly prescribe tricyclic anti-depressants, benzodiazepines, among others (C. Wright, FDA, personal communication, 1994).

[b]Categories are not mutually exclusive; patients are counted in any of 10 combined categories of drugs, depending on mentions of the drug in the discharge records.

[c]Includes crack cocaine.

[d]The first percentage refers to the residential setting and the second refers to the hospital inpatient setting.

[e]Figure refers to residential setting rather than treatment modality because there is no separate breakdown for chemical dependency programs or therapeutic communities (in Table 30, Batten et al., 1992).

[f]Figure refers to hospital inpatient setting rather than modality because there is no separate listing for hospital-based chemical dependency programs (in Table 30, Batten et al., 1992).

SOURCES: IOM, 1990; Batten et al., 1992.

Methadone maintenance programs, although geared toward opiate-dependent patients, have witnessed an increase in patients who are poly-drug users. About 39 percent of patients in methadone maintenance programs report having used cocaine prior to treatment (Batten et al., 1992). While in methadone treatment, cocaine use varies widely. A recent review article (Condelli et al., 1991) cites several studies that have documented concomitant cocaine use in as few as 16 percent and as many as 75 percent of methadone patients. One study, conducted by the General Accounting Office (GAO, 1990) found cocaine use to occur in more than 20 percent of patients in more than one-third of the methadone programs under study. Some methadone programs do not provide any additional services for cocaine users; others have instituted behavioral interventions such as rewarding patients who cease cocaine use with additional methadone take-home doses (Condelli et al., 1991).

Therapeutic communities are highly structured long-term residential programs tailored primarily to the hard-core user. Over the 9 to 12 months of treatment, therapeutic communities emphasize complete abstinence from drug use and other changes in lifestyle. The philosophy is to create a productive, alternative environment for those whose addiction has led to criminal and anti-social behavior. The staff are mostly recovered drug-users. Most TCs are strongly opposed to pharmacotherapy of any kind. Only 5.6 percent of patients receive treatment in long-term TC programs (U.S. DHHS, 1993).

Chemical dependency programs are mostly short-term residential programs that were developed for alcoholics. They use the 12-step model of Alcoholics Anonymous to facilitate recovery. With the surge in cocaine use in the 1980s, more than one-half of the patients in chemical dependency programs were cocaine users (Rawson et al., 1991). The treatment model developed for alcoholism was applied to cocaine dependence with little modification. The goal is complete abstinence accompanied by lifestyle change. Intensive counseling is often provided by psychologists, psychiatrists, and recovered drug users. Even though the emphasis of treatment is on counseling, prescription drugs such as anti-depressants and benzodiazepines are often used. In the 1980s, CD programs were often found in hospitals, but the cost of a typical 28-day stay was so prohibitive that insurers began to restrict coverage for hospital-based CD programs. Consequently, most CD programs have been moved to residential settings (Rawson et al., 1991), and they are generally the treatment of choice for patients who have private insurance (IOM, 1990).

DEMOGRAPHIC AND FINANCIAL PROFILE

The separation of opiate- and cocaine-dependent populations must be understood as somewhat artificial because poly-drug use has become the norm (McLellan et al., in press). Nevertheless, researchers and practitioners recognize that many persons who are dependent on drugs have a clearly defined preference for a particular drug, as defined by the duration and intensity of past use. This drug is often referred to as the primary drug of abuse. Therefore, whenever this chapter refers to an "opiate-dependent" or a "cocaine-dependent" patient, it should be understood that this assignation refers to the primary drug.

It must be underscored that the demographic and financial data presented here concerns patients in specialty treatment programs, those programs dedicated to drug-abuse treatment in free-standing clinics or in a specialized wing of a hospital. Similar data are not available for patients who receive treatment in nonspecialty settings.

Opiate-Dependent Patients

There are an estimated 1 million regular users of illicit opiates and an estimated 500,000 opiate-addicted individuals in the United States (Kreek, 1992). Only a fraction of opiate-dependent patients—an estimated 117,000 patients—received methadone maintenance treatment in 1993 (Harwood et al., 1994). That point is relevant for the pharmaceutical industry, as they are interested in the two subsets of opiate addicts: those currently in treatment, and those who might come in for treatment if other pharmacologic modalities were available. The demographics of opiate-dependent patients in methadone maintenance programs are presented in Table 4.2. Much of these data are drawn from national or nationally representative data sets—NDATUS, the Client Data System (CDS)[3] (SAMHSA, 1994), and the Drug Services Research Survey[4] (Batten et al., 1992; 1993). Almost 50 percent of patients are located in New York and California (U.S. DHHS, 1993). About 67 percent of methadone patients are male (SAMHSA, 1994).

Methadone patients are somewhat older than are cocaine-dependent patients in drug treatment. Almost 23 percent of methadone patients are ages 20–29, and another 75 percent are over age 30. By comparison, 44 percent of cocaine-dependent patients are ages 20–25, and 51.5 percent are over age 30 (SAMHSA, 1994). Employment indicators reveal that almost half of methadone patients are not in the labor force, about 32 percent are unemployed, and only 24 percent are employed part or full time (SAMHSA, 1994). There are no nationwide data on

---

[3]The Client Data System (CDS) is an annual and voluntary reporting system on admissions to specialty substance abuse treatment programs throughout the United States. Most of the programs receive some public funds. The 1992 CDS contains information for 40 states, the District of Columbia, and Puerto Rico, covering 89 percent of the U.S. population.

[4]The Drug Services Research Survey (DSRS) was conducted in two phases—a nationally representative sample of drug treatment facilities (Phase I) and a survey of client discharge records (Phase II). The objective was to gather data on the characteristics of drug treatment facilities, clients in treatment, and financing. Phase I collected data from treatment facilities for the point prevalence date of March 30, 1990, and for their most recent 12-month reporting period. Phase II examined a sample of the records of 2,182 clients discharged from treatment facilities during the 12 months between September 1, 1989, and August 31, 1990.

methadone patient income levels. Yet one large study of 22 publicly and privately funded programs found that opiate-dependent patients (N = 195) had an average income of $417 in the 30 days before treatment (McLellan et al., in press). Taken together, the employment and income data support the commonly held view that most methadone patients are indigent.

TABLE 4.2 Demographics of Methadone and Cocaine-Dependent Patients in Treatment[1]

Characteristics	Methadone Patients	Cocaine-Dependent Patients
Patients in treatment, 1993	117,000[2,c]	300,000–400,000[3]
Admissions, 1992[d]	112,016	385,699
Age[d]		
20–24 years	7.6%	16.0%
25–29 years	15.2%	27.7%
30–34 years	22.5%	27.0%
35–44 years	41.6%	21.2%
45+ years	11.1%	3.3%
Male[d]	66.5%	66.6%
Married	22%[g]	22–32%[6]
Employment status[d]		
Not employed	31.6%	31.8%
Employed full-time	18.2%	19.7%
Employed part-time	5.6%	5.4%
Not in labor force	44.6%	43.1%
Average income		
30 days prior to treatment	$417[a]	$613[a]
Annual	NA	$24,000[7]
Length of stay in days[g]	321	109[8]
Health insurance[4,d]		
None	49.4%	53.9%
Medicaid	16.5%	11.0%
Private insurance	4.2%	5.1%
Blue Cross/Blue Shield	3.2%	2.8%
Medicare	1.5%	0.8%
HMO	1.8%	1.7%
Unknown	21.1%	22.4%

TABLE 4.2 Continued

Characteristics	Methadone Patients	Cocaine-Dependent Patients
Primary source of payment at admission[5,d]		
Private health insurance	5.2%	6.8%
Medicaid	15.4%	11.7%
Client fees (self-pay)	21.5%	20.1%
Unknown	22.0%	20.3%

[1]The patient populations in this table are divided according to primary drug of abuse.
[2]Extrapolation from NDATUS 1991 point prevalence of 95,286 patients in treatment by Harwood and co-workers (1994).
[3]Assumes 30–40 percent of the estimated 1 million patients in treatment in 1993 (Harwood et al., 1994) are primarily dependent on cocaine or crack.
[4]In the CDS, health insurance information is collected irrespective of whether it covers the current treatment episode. Health insurance status is an optional data item reported by 21 states and jurisdictions, covering 42 percent of the U.S. population (SAMHSA, 1994).
[5]This information refers to the treatment episode in which the data were collected. Primary source of payment is an optional data item reported by 17 states and jurisdictions, covering 19 percent of the U.S. population (SAMHSA, 1994).
[6]Ranges were compiled from three studies with large, but not necessarily nationally representative, samples (McLellan et al., in press; Rawson et al., 1993; Means et al., 1989).
[7]Average income from sample studied 1986–1989, unadjusted for inflation (Rawson et al., 1993).
[8]Figure refers to *all* patients in a nationally representative sample of drug and alcohol treatment programs, irrespective of primary drug of abuse. Breakdowns for cocaine-dependent patients are not available from the published report. The figure of 109 days averages hospital inpatients (23.9 days), residential patients (47.4 days), and ODF (177.9 days), among other modalities (Batten et al., 1992).

SOURCES: McLellan et al., in press[a]; Butynski et al., 1994[b]; Harwood et al., 1994[c]; SAMHSA, 1994[d]; Rawson et al., 1993[e]; U.S. DHHS, 1993[f]; Batten et al., 1992[g]; Means et al., 1989[h].

Very few patients have private health insurance, and even fewer use their insurance to pay for treatment. According to the 1992 Client Data System (CDS) 9.2 percent of patients have private insurance, but only 5.2 percent of patients list it as the expected source of payment at the time of admission to treatment.[5] About 15.4 percent of patients list Medicaid as the expected source of payment. Many of the remaining patients—about 21.5 percent—plan to pay for their own treatment (SAMHSA, 1994). It is surprising that so few patients have or use private health insurance to pay for treatment, given that almost one-quarter of patients are employed. Privately insured patients might be afraid to report or to take advantage of their coverage because they fear employer notification or their policies may be overly restrictive.[6] The dearth of insured patients is underscored by financing data presented in Chapter 5. Those data show that private insurance accounts for 2.5 percent and 11.5 percent of methadone and cocaine treatment financing, respectively.

Methadone maintenance treatment is considered long-term. The average length of stay—the time from admission to discharge—is 320 days, yet owing to wide variability, the median length of stay is 4.5 months (Batten et al., 1992). Some patients remain in treatment indefinitely; others eventually reduce their methadone doses to abstinence, thereby concluding treatment. Attesting to the chronic, relapsing nature of opiate addiction is the finding that almost 80 percent of methadone patients admitted to and discharged from treatment have had prior treatment episodes. Those patients average 3.4 previous treatment episodes, 1.4 of which occurred in the prior year (Batten et al., 1992).

Cocaine-Dependent Patients

The primary source of nationwide data on the demographic characteristics of cocaine-dependent patients admitted to treatment is the Client Data System (CDS) sponsored by the Substance Abuse and Mental Health Services Administration (SAMHSA) (1994). Other national or nationally representative data bases generally do not stratify the data by drug of abuse.

Because CDS is based on admissions—admissions are usually higher than the number of clients in treatment because clients are often readmitted to treatment in the same year—it does not contain estimates of the number of patients in treatment. Yet it can be reasonably estimated that the number of patients in treatment in 1993 was 300,000–400,000. That figure assumes 30–40

---

[5]Data items on health insurance coverage in general (regardless of whether it is used) and on the primary source of payment for a treatment admission are optional and reported by 21 and 17 states and jurisdictions, respectively, covering 42 percent and 19 percent of the U.S. population.

[6]Restrictions take the form of preexisting condition limitations and limits on the number of inpatient days, outpatient visits, or both (Chapter 5).

percent of the estimated 1 million patients in treatment in 1993 (Harwood et al., 1994) used cocaine before entering treatment. That assumption is partly based on the Drug Services Research Survey (DSRS), which found that 31 percent of all patients in treatment report having used cocaine or crack in the 30 days before admission (Batten et al., 1992). DSRS was conducted in 1990, and since that time there is evidence that the percentage of cocaine-dependent patients in treatment is increasing. Butynski and co-workers (1994) report that admissions to cocaine addiction treatment programs escalated from 18.9 percent in 1987 to 36.1 percent in 1990 then reached 44.8 percent of all treatment admissions in 1992. The rise in cocaine admissionⱼ could reflect, among other factors, increased cocaine consumption by heavy users, especially of crack cocaine (Gfroerer and Brodsky, 1993). Over the past decade, there has been a decline in the number of light users, yet no decline in the number of heavy users (Rydell and Everingham, 1994).

Cocaine-dependent patients also frequently use alcohol and marijuana (Washton, 1990; Rawson et al., 1993; McLellan et al., in press). The consumption of alcohol and the smoking of marijuana help to ameliorate the intense stimulant effect of high-dose cocaine (Washton, 1990).

In comparison with methadone patients, cocaine-dependent patients tend to be somewhat younger and have shorter lengths of stay in treatment (Table 4.2). Apart from these differences, the opiate- and cocaine-dependent patient populations are very similar (although it must be remembered that CDS data are biased in favor of publicly funded programs). Sex, marital status, employment, and health insurance indicators are quite similar. One of the only differences is that fewer cocaine-dependent patients are either insured by or use Medicaid.

Income levels are not reported in national surveys partly because of the difficulty in obtaining accurate information from patients who might have illegal income. The income data presented in Table 4.2 are compiled from large, but not necessarily nationally representative, studies. In one of those studies, cocaine-dependent patients enrolled in 22 publicly and privately funded programs in the Philadelphia area reported earnings from the 30 days before admission that were 32 percent higher than were earnings for opiate-dependent patients (McLellan et al., in press). Annual income of patients in treatment has been reported in two studies, both of which pertain to cocaine. Rawson and co-workers (1993) found a mean legal annual income of $24,000 among a sample of 486 patients entering cocaine addiction treatment programs in Los Angeles between 1986 and 1989. That figure averages patient groups at two clinics, one of which was located in affluent Beverly Hills and the other in a low-income area in San Bernardino County. A smaller study of 81 outpatients in treatment in New York between 1985 and 1986 revealed that 53 percent reported incomes of less than $25,000, 16 percent reported incomes above $25,000; and 30 percent did not report income (Means et al., 1989). Those studies collectively suggest that cocaine-dependent patients could be financially better off than opiate-dependent patients, but it is unknown whether the data are nationally representative or reflective of current patients. The epidemic of cocaine use among the upper and middle classes in the mid-1980s appears to have abated, only to be replaced by an increase in dependence on the more affordable and more dangerous crack cocaine among lower income users (Rawson et al., 1991).

Of those factors, inadequate dosing and inadequate time in treatment have received much attention as reasons for treatment failure (IOM, 1990). D'Aunno and Vaughn (1992) found that 33 percent of treatment programs in a nationally random sample of 172 methadone treatment programs administered average doses of 41–50 milligrams, and 34 percent administered doses between 10–40 milligrams—amounts that are below the recommended dose of at least 60 milligrams (NIDA, 1989). Low dosage, as mandated by some states, recommended by others, is countertherapeutic. When higher doses are administered, patients have longer average lengths of time in treatment, which is by itself an independent predictor of better treatment outcomes (IOM, 1990; Prendergast et al., in press). For example, in a randomized, double-blind, placebo-controlled study, patients who received the highest dose of methadone had better retention in treatment than did those who received lower doses. Those same patients also had the greatest reductions in opiate and cocaine use while in treatment (Strain et al., 1993).

TREATMENT EFFECTIVENESS AND COST-EFFECTIVENESS

Methadone Maintenance Treatment

Effectiveness

There is strong consensus that methadone maintenance treatment is effective for the treatment of opiate addiction (IOM, 1990; OTA, 1990; Anglin and Hser, 1992; Prendergast et al., in press). The results of a large body of research reveal that treatment works; patients fare better during and long after treatment than before treatment. They also have better outcomes than do those who are untreated, those who are on waiting lists for treatment, and those who are simply detoxified with methadone. The best measure of treatment effectiveness is reduced opiate use. Other measures are reduced use of alcohol and other drugs, reduced criminal activity, reduced intravenous drug use, and reduced health care costs. When relapse to opiate use does occur after treatment, it should be interpreted as a reflection of the chronic and relapsing nature of addiction, the quality of treatment, or patient characteristics (Tims et al., 1991; McLellan et al., in press).

An important study by McLellan and co-workers (1993) confirms the effectiveness of methadone maintenance by revealing the critical role of counseling and rehabilitative services offered along with pharmacotherapy. The study employs random assignment to treatment groups, thereby overcoming some of the problems plaguing earlier research, which used naturalistic settings and patient self-assignments (Tims et al., 1991). After assigning patients to three different groups with varying levels of care, McLellan and co-workers found that patients given methadone and a comprehensive array of treatment services had significantly better treatment outcomes than did those who were given methadone and counseling, and than did those given methadone alone. Figure 4.2 illustrates the benefits of comprehensive treatment in reducing opiate usage over 16 weeks of treatment. After this intensive treatment regimen, patients sometimes require less counseling to succeed in treatment (T. McLellan, University of Pennsylvania, personal communication, 1994).

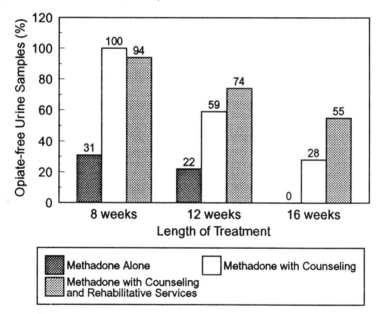

FIGURE 4.2 Effectiveness of methadone with counseling and rehabilitative services. SOURCE: McLellan et al., 1993.

Unfortunately, the real world of treatment stands in sharp contrast to the research setting. There is great variability in the effectiveness of treatment (Ball and Ross, 1991). For instance, GAO (1990) found that at 10 of 24 treatment programs, a range of 21–47 percent of patients were using heroin after 6 months of treatment. The variability in outcomes can be attributed to many factors, including inadequate dosing, length of time in treatment, program policies, staff quality, and patient characteristics (e.g., severity of the problem, health and insurance status, and patient compliance with treatment).

Cost-Effectiveness[7]

Current estimates used in Figure 4.3 place the average cost per methadone admission to a treatment program at $1,390 (Harwood et al., 1994). Those costs are not dissimilar to those from a decade ago when a large study of methadone's cost-effectiveness was conducted.[8] The Treatment Outcome Prospective Study (TOPS) followed 11,000 patients in 41 treatment programs nationwide (Harwood et al., 1988; Hubbard et al., 1989). The investigators compared the cost of treatment with the benefits from reduced criminal activity during treatment and one year after treatment. They found that the ratio of benefits-to-costs was 4 to 1, when they defined the benefits in terms of reduced costs to victims, reduced criminal justice costs, and reduced losses owing to theft. Those benefits were described collectively as the benefits to "law-abiding citizens" because they included benefits that were only realized by the victims. The benefit-to-cost ratio was not as robust, using a broader measure of overall societal benefits (Hubbard et al., 1989). That second measure included the societal benefit of enhanced legitimate earnings by the drug abuser following treatment. Since drug abusers' earnings were not found to increase after treatment, overall societal benefits were not as great as the benefits to-law abiding citizens.[9] There is strong evidence

---

[7]In this chapter, the terms "cost-effectiveness" and "cost-benefit" are used synonymously. Technically, cost-effectiveness is the relationship between program costs, which are measured in dollars, and program effects, which are measured in other units. Cost-benefit analysis is the relationship between program costs and the benefits, both measured in dollars (Apsler and Harding, 1991).

[8]The National Institute on Drug Abuse (NIDA) is currently conducting the Drug Abuse Treatment Outcome Study, under contract with Research Triangle Institute. This is a multiyear, longitudinal study of 10,000 adult clients in 80 of the best treatment programs in 12 cities. In addition, SAMHSA is supporting the Services Research Outcomes Study on a cohort of clients after treatment for substance abuse. The analysis will focus on treatment outcomes in relation to provider and staff characteristics and to the costs of treatment.

[9]The benefits to "law-abiding" citizens is a measure defined by the study authors to emphasize benefits which are experienced by the victims and their families, such as reduced losses from property or money stolen during a crime. By contrast, there is no net benefit to society—the other benefit measure—when theft takes place, because the value of the stolen goods is transferred from the law-abiding citizen to the criminal.

from research on alcohol dependence that treatment can significantly reduce overall medical costs (Holder and Blose, 1992), but until recently, there has been only limited research on the medical offsets of treatment for drug dependence.

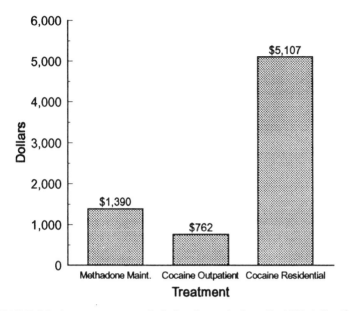

FIGURE 4.3 Average cost per admission for methadone (in 1993 dollars)[a] and cocaine treatment (in 1992 dollars)[b]. SOURCES: Harwood et al., 1994[a]; Rydell and Everingham, 1994[b].

A new study of cost-effectiveness in the state of California was published in July 1994 (Gerstein et al., 1994). The California Drug and Alcohol Treatment Assessment (CALDATA) analyzed the consequences of four treatment modalities, including methadone maintenance, on a random sample of 3,000 patients in treatment or discharged in fiscal year (FY) 1992. The sample was designed to represent almost 150,000 patients in treatment programs throughout the state. It was the first to compare the cost of treatment with the economic benefits not only in crime reduction and productivity, but also in health care use. The analysis used two separate benefit measures, similar to those in TOPS (i.e., the benefits to tax-paying citizens and the benefits to society)[10] but incorporated measures of health care use. Study subjects were interviewed an average of 15

---

[10]CALDATA measured benefits in terms of avoiding costs to tax-paying citizens and avoiding costs to society. However, for clarity these terms are referred to here as benefits to tax-paying citizens and benefits to society.

months after treatment and asked to recall the frequency of criminal, health, and productivity characteristics and behaviors before, during, and after treatment. By assigning monetary values to those characteristics and behaviors, researchers were able to calculate savings (or benefits) during and after treatment by comparison with the year before treatment.

The overall benefit-to-cost ratio to taxpayers from all treatment modalities was 7.1 to 1. That was higher than the benefit-to-cost ratio to society (2.2 to 1). For methadone treatment, the analysis was stratified by methadone patients discharged from treatment and those continuing in treatment. Methadone patients continuing in treatment are long-term patients who were still in treatment at the time CALDATA was conducted. The percentage of discharged patients who used heroin declined by 46.5 percent in comparison to before treatment. Health care expenditures for methadone discharges—measured in terms of emergency room use and outpatient and inpatient health and mental health care—declined by 20.6 percent. Their legitimate earnings after treatment decreased by 33 percent, a finding that suggested to the authors that the short period of treatment was unsuccessful at helping them become gainfully employed. Health care expenditures for methadone patients who continued in treatment declined by 12.6 percent in comparison to before treatment. For this same group, legitimate earnings increased during treatment by about 10 percent.

When all the benefit and cost measures were taken into account for each category of methadone patient, the ratio was favorable. The benefit-to-cost ratio was 12.6 to 1 for discharged methadone patients and 4.8 to 1 for methadone patients continuing in treatment, when the benefits were measured for taxpayers. The benefit-to-cost ratio was –3 to 1 and 4.7 to 1, respectively, when the more conservative measure of benefits to society was analyzed.

One final point bears emphasis. It is often noted that treatment is far less costly than alternatives such as untreated addiction, incarceration and parole. Supporting this commonly held view, Figure 4.4 compares the annual cost of treatment with these alternatives. To lend empirical support, Deschenes and co-workers (1991) studied the careers of about 300 heroin-dependent persons before and during treatment. The annual cost per person for arrests, incarceration, and parole dropped by about half (from about $8,000–$9,000 to about $4,000) when active addiction ceased and treatment began.

Cocaine Addiction Treatment

Effectiveness

A variety of outpatient and residential treatments are available for cocaine addiction, most of which offer counseling in the form of group and individual therapy. Although there is some prescribing of medications to help achieve abstinence and prevent relapse, none of the available medications are effective in consistently reducing return to cocaine use (Chapter 2). An accumulating body of research points to some effectiveness for specific types of cocaine addiction treatment and to better outcomes for patients who remain in treatment longer (IOM, 1990; Prendergast et al., in press). However, there is no consensus about the most effective treatment modality for cocaine addiction (Leukefeld and Tims, 1993; Carroll et al., 1994). The problem is that much of the research has focused on individual treatment modalities rather than on the comparative efficacy of different modalities. The study designs typically compare pre- to post-treatment gains in abstinence. When studies are conducted to make comparisons across modalities, patients are randomly assigned to one modality. Although this is the best method for accurate comparison, it often results in the majority of patients dropping out of the assigned treatment.

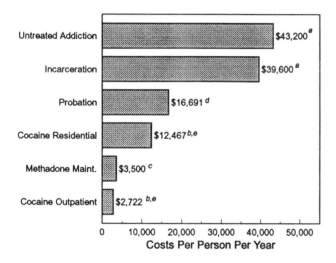

FIGURE 4.4 Treatment is less expensive than alternatives. NOTE: [a]1991 dollars; [b]1992 dollars; [c]1993 dollars; [d]1992 dollars, inflation adjusted from 1983 data; [e]The average cost per admission is much lower than this figure because most patients are in treatment less than 1 year. SOURCES: McLellan et al., 1994; Lewin-VHI, unpublished estimates; Rydell and Everingham, 1994; SAMHSA, 1994.

There is growing awareness that no one treatment will work for everyone who is dependent on cocaine, and the choice of treatment could be dictated by the severity of addiction. In general, addiction treatment professionals support initial evaluation and case management to ensure that patients with more severe conditions are treated in settings with the highest intensity of services (such as residential settings) and that those with less severe addictions are treated in outpatient settings (ASAM, 1990; CASA, 1993).

TOPS is the largest and most frequently cited study of cocaine addiction treatment effectiveness (Hubbard et al., 1989). For patients who remained in treatment 3 months or longer, somewhat less than half were abstinent 1 year after treatment. Among residential patients—all of whom were in TCs—the prevalence of regular cocaine use declined from 28 percent before treatment to 16 percent one year after; among outpatient drug-free patients, the prevalence declined from 13 percent to 8 percent; and among outpatient methadone patients, the prevalence declined from 26 percent to 17 percent. The authors guard against strict comparisons across modalities because of patient self-selection to treatment and because of patient and program heterogeneity. TOPS did not examine the effectiveness of chemical dependency programs. Prendergast and colleagues (in press) observe that there are no well-designed studies of CD programs, but there are some limited studies showing treatment effectiveness.

A study of 300 cocaine dependent males entering the West Los Angeles Veterans Administration Medical Center for inpatient, outpatient, or self-help programs found abstinence at the 12-month follow-up to be greatest among patients whose choice of treatment consisted of an initial 21-day inpatient period, an outpatient follow-up regimen, and continued involvement in self-help groups (Khalsa and Anglin, 1991). A newer study of 649 drug-dependent patients admitted to 22 public and private programs—both inpatient and outpatient—in the Philadelphia area has found that, of the 212 cocaine-dependent patients entering treatment, 51 percent were abstinent from all illicit drugs at the follow-up interview 6 months after entering treatment (McLellan et al., 1994; in press). The study subjects included all patients who completed at least 5 inpatient days or at least two consecutive outpatient treatment sessions. Improvements also were found in measures of psychiatric, employment, and family status in addition to measures of improved public health and safety. For all study subjects, including cocaine, opiate, and alcohol patients, the degree of drug use at the 6-month follow-up was predicted by the greater severity of the drug abuse problem at the time of admission. The type of treatment—the number of psychosocial services such as psychotherapy, family therapy, and employment counseling—was not related to post-treatment drug use, but it was related to psychosocial adjustment after treatment. When stratifying that data and some additional data by whether the program was funded privately or publicly, it was found that private patients, all of whom were insured, were far healthier and had more resources as they entered treatment, received more services in treatment, and experienced 20–40 percent more improvement than did patients in publicly funded programs (Weisner and McLellan, 1994).

Newer studies of cocaine addiction treatment effectiveness also have focused on particular types of structured outpatient programs. Encouraging findings from intensive outpatient programs have been reported by Washton and co-workers (Washton, 1990; Washton and Stone-Washton, 1993). Using a neurobehavioral model, Rawson and co-workers (1993) reported that 40–44 percent of patients who completed 6 months of treatment attained abstinence during an open trial, a finding they hope to replicate in a randomized trial that is under way. Another treatment that deserves attention has been pioneered by Higgins and co-workers. Their outpatient regimen is a behavioral approach using contingency management procedures (Higgins et al., 1991; 1993). That technique adapts the principles of operant conditioning to the treatment of cocaine abuse. Patients who remain abstinent during treatment accumulate vouchers of increasing value the longer they remain abstinent. The vouchers are worth up to about $1,000 over 12 weeks of treatment and can be used to purchase items selected by the patient and purchased by the counselor. The most recent study using random assignment to treatment groups found this behavioral approach superior to counseling in patient retention and abstinence (Higgins et al., 1993).

Cost-Effectiveness

The average cost of an outpatient admission for cocaine addiction treatment, presented in Figure 4.3, is estimated at $762; the average cost of a residential admission is estimated at $5,107 (Rydell and Everingham, 1994). Several major studies of cost-effectiveness have been undertaken. TOPS studied the cost of treatment in comparison to the benefits in crime reduction, as discussed earlier. The ratio of benefits to costs for each of the three treatment modalities studied (outpatient methadone, residential, outpatient drug-free) ranged from about 4 to 1 to about 1 to 1, depending on the modality and the benefit measure used. Even though this analysis focused on all of the patients in a given treatment modality, rather than on cocaine-addicted patients per se, the findings are relevant because cocaine use was found to varying degrees among patients in all three treatment modalities and was shown to decline from pretreatment levels.

A new study from California (CALDATA), cited earlier, also analyzed the cost-benefits of residential and outpatient drug-free treatment modalities (Gerstein et al., 1994). Cocaine was the primary drug of abuse in 29 percent of residential and 32 percent of outpatient drug-free (ODF) patients. The percentage of patients using cocaine in all treatment modalities declined by about 46 percent after treatment, pointing to treatment effectiveness. Favorable benefit-to-cost ratios were found, yet they varied according to treatment modality and the method used to assess benefits. For tax-paying citizens, the ratio of benefits-to-costs of treatment was 4.8 to 1 for residential patients and 11 to 1 for ODF patients. In terms of benefits to society, the ratio was 2.4 to 1 and 2.9 to 1, respectively.

There is a recent, two-volume RAND study demonstrating the relative cost-effectiveness of treatment (Everingham and Rydell, 1994; Rydell and Everingham, 1994). Treatment was found to surpass all other societal control strategies in terms of relative cost-effectiveness. The study compared treatment (a demand control strategy) and three supply control strategies: source country control, interdiction, and domestic enforcement (cocaine seizures, arrests, and imprisonment of drug dealers). It calculated the cost required for each control strategy to achieve a common measure of effectiveness—a reduction in cocaine consumption by 1 percent of current annual consumption. To meet this objective, researchers found that the additional cost of treatment would be $34 million, an amount 7.3 times less than that needed for the next most effective strategy, domestic enforcement, and 23 times less expensive than source control (Figure 4.5). The researchers conclude, "Our findings suggest a way to make cocaine control policy more cost-effective: cut back on supply control programs and expand treatment of heavy users," (Rydell and Everingham, 1994).

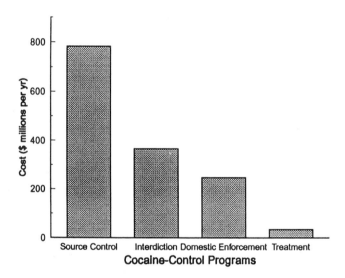

FIGURE 4.5 Additional cost of reducing cocaine consumption by 1% with alternative cocaine-control programs. Treatment is the most cost-effective approach to reducing cocaine consumption. It is 7.3 times less costly than the least expensive alternative, domestic enforcement, and 23 times less costly than source control. SOURCE: Rydell and Everingham, 1994.

In the years ahead, even in the absence of a new medication, cocaine addiction treatment is likely to become even more cost-effective. Managed care, case management, and other medical cost containment approaches, which are discussed in Chapter 5, are being used to shift patients from the inpatient to the outpatient setting. For example, Alterman and co-workers (1994) have found intensive day treatment to be as effective as and less expensive than inpatient treatment for cocaine addiction. Reductions in average treatment costs not only enhance the absolute cost-effectiveness of treatment, but they also increase the cost-effectiveness of treatment relative to other control strategies. Were a new and effective medication for cocaine addiction treatment to become available, treatment costs[11] could be reduced even further, through reduced counseling costs. That already has been demonstrated in the mental health field with the introduction of lithium for manic depression and clozapine for schizophrenia (Wyatt and de Saint Ghislain, in press). For example, savings of $1 billion per year (in 1991 dollars) in direct inpatient and outpatient costs have been realized since the marketing of lithium in 1970. A new cocaine medication does hold the opportunity to reduce some, but not all, of the counseling costs, as some degree of counseling, along with pharmacotherapy, as essential ingredients of cocaine addiction treatment will continue to be necessary, as research on methadone maintenance suggests (McLellan et al., 1993).

CONCLUSIONS AND RECOMMENDATION

Effective pharmacotherapies are currently marketed for opiate addiction, but not for cocaine addiction. Current treatment strategies for cocaine addiction depend mostly on a variety of counseling approaches undertaken in residential or outpatient settings. The opiate- and cocaine-dependent patient populations are similar, except with respect to age and length of stay in treatment. Cocaine-dependent patients tend to be younger and have shorter term treatment episodes.

Unemployment and a lack of private health insurance are common among the opiate- and cocaine-dependent patient populations. About 10 percent have private insurance; an even smaller fraction appear to use their coverage to pay for an episode of treatment. Cocaine-dependent patients seem to have greater income than do opiate-dependent patients, but the evidence is not conclusive. Cocaine-dependent patients are perceived to have incomes higher than those of methadone patients, but this perception could be outdated because cocaine use, since the mid-1980s, appears to have declined among the middle and upper classes. Lack of insurance and insufficient patient resources to pay for treatment are frequently cited by the pharmaceutical industry as deterrents to pharmaceutical investment.

---

[11]The current average cost per cocaine admission of $1,740. This figure is a weighted average of outpatient and residential treatment (Rydell and Everingham, 1994).

There is resounding evidence of treatment effectiveness for methadone maintenance. Treatment is effective in reducing opiate use, criminal activity, and intravenous drug use. The evidence of treatment effectiveness is not as strong for cocaine, yet there is an accumulating body of research pointing to the effectiveness of psychosocial treatment modalities. As yet, there is not a pharmacologic agent for the treatment of cocaine addiction or a medication to reduce cocaine craving.

Treatments for opiate and cocaine addiction are cost-effective. When the cost of opiate- and cocaine-addiction treatment is compared to the benefits in reduced crime, the result is unambiguous: every dollar invested in treatment yields two and up to four dollars, and sometimes more, in societal benefits. Treatment also averts other health care costs. In short, current treatments for opiate and cocaine addiction, although variable in nature and cost, are effective and cost-effective. Clearly the federal government should make every effort to expand the treatment capabilities of the states. New medications, especially for cocaine addiction, do hold the potential to reduce some of the need for counseling, which forms the largest share of treatment charges. With lower overall treatment costs, treatment can prove to become even more cost-effective.

Given the data presented on the effectiveness and cost-effectiveness of both opiate- and cocaine-addiction treatment, and in light of the evidence that treatment is far more cost-effective than are other control strategies, such as domestic enforcement, interdiction, and source country control, the federal government should make treatment a major component of its drug control strategies.

The committee strongly recommends expanding the treatment capabilities of the states for opiate- and cocaine-dependent individuals to ensure that all those seeking treatment obtain it without delay. The recommendation may be implemented by:

•   Providing additional money to increase treatment in states where there are waiting lists.
•   Shifting money from supply control programs to treatment programs.

REFERENCES

Alterman AI, O'Brien CP, McLellan AT, August DS, Snider EC, Droba M, Cornish JW, Hall CP, Raphaelson AH, Schrade FX. 1994. Effectiveness and costs of inpatient versus day hospital cocaine rehabilitation. Journal of Nervous and Mental Disorders 182:157–163.

Anglin MD, Hser Y. 1992. Treatment of drug abuse. In: Watson RW, ed. Drug Abuse Treatment. New York: Humana Press. Vol. 3, Drug and Alcohol Abuse Reviews.

Apsler R, Harding WM. 1991. Cost-effectiveness analysis of drug abuse treatment: current status and recommendations for future research. In: NIDA Drug Abuse Services Research Series, No. 1. 58–81.

ASAM (American Society of Addiction Medicine), Inc. 1990. Public Policy Statement on Managed Care and Addiction Medicine. Adopted by ASAM Board of Directors, November 1990.

Ball JC, Ross A. 1991. The Effectiveness of Methadone Maintenance Treatment. New York: Springer-Verlag.

Batten H, Prottas J, Horgan CM, Simon LJ, Larson MJ, Elliott EA, Marsden ME. 1992. Drug Services Research Survey Final Report: Phase II. Waltham, MA: Bigel Institute for Health Policy, Brandeis University. Contract number 271-90-8319/1. Submitted to the National Institute of Drug Abuse, February 12, 1992.

Batten H, Horgan CM, Prottas J, Simon LJ, Larson MJ, Elliott EA, Bowden ML, Lee M. 1993. Drug Services Research Survey Final Report: Phase I. Waltham, MA: Bigel Institute for Health Policy, Brandeis University. Contract number 271-90-8319/1. Submitted to the National Institute of Drug Abuse, February 22, 1993.

Butynski W, Reda J, Bartosch W, McMullen H, Nelson S, Anderson R, Ciaccio M, Sheehan K, Fitzgerald C. 1994. State Resources and Services Related to Alcohol and Other Drug Problems for Fiscal Year 1992. Washington, DC: National Association of State Alcohol and Drug Abuse Directors, Inc.

Carroll KM, Rounsaville BJ, Gordon LT, Nich C, Jatlow P, Bisighini RM, Gawin FH. 1994. Psychotherapy and pharmacotherapy for ambulatory cocaine abusers. Archives of General Psychiatry 51:177–187.

CASA (Center on Addiction and Substance Abuse). 1993. Recommendations on Substance Abuse Coverage and Health Care Reform. New York: Center on Addiction and Substance Abuse at Columbia University in collaboration with the Brown University Center for Alcohol and Addiction Studies.

Condelli WS, Fairbank JA, Dennis ML, Rachal JV. 1991. Cocaine use by clients in methadone programs: significance, scope, and behavioral interventions. Journal of Substance Abuse Treatment 8:203–212.

D'Aunno T, Vaughn TE. 1992. Variation in methadone treatment practices. Journal of the American Medical Association 267:253–258.

Deschenes EP, Anglin MD, Speckart G. 1991. Narcotic addiction: related criminal careers, social and economic costs. Journal of Drug Issues 21:383–411.

Everingham S, Rydell C. 1994. Modeling the Demand for Cocaine. Santa Monica, CA: RAND Drug Policy Research Center. MR-332-ONDCP/A/DPRC.

Federal Register. 1989. Food and Drug Administration, National Institute on Drug Abuse, Methadone in Maintenance and Detoxification; Joint Revision of Conditions for Use (final rule). 54: 8954.

GAO (General Accounting Office). 1990. Methadone Maintenance: Some Treatment Programs Are Not Effective: Greater Federal Oversight Needed. Washington, DC: GAO. GAO/HRD-90-104.

Gerstein DR, Johnson RA, Harwood HJ, Fountain D, Suter N, Malloy K. 1994. Evaluating Recovery Services: The California Drug and Alcohol Treatment

Assessment (CALDATA). Sacramento, CA: California Department of Alcohol and Drug Programs.

Gfroerer JC, Brodsky MD. 1993. Frequent cocaine users and their use of treatment. American Journal of Public Health 83:1149–1154.

Harwood HJ, Hubbard RL, Collins JJ, Rachal JV. 1988. The costs of crime and the benefits of drug abuse treatment: a cost-benefit analysis using TOPS data. In: Leukefeld CG, Tims FM, eds. Compulsory Treatment of Drug Abuse: Research and Clinical Practice. (NIDA Research Monograph 86:209–235). Rockville, MD: NIDA.

Harwood HJ, Thomsom M, Nesmith T. 1994. Healthcare Reform and Substance Abuse Treatment: The Cost of Financing Under Alternative Approaches. Fairfax, VA: Lewin-VHI.

Higgins ST, Delany DD, Budney AJ, Bickel WK, Hughes JR, Foerg F, Fenwick JW. 1991. A behavioral approach to achieving initial cocaine abstinence. American Journal of Psychiatry 148:1218–1224.

Higgins ST, Budney AJ, Bickel WK, Hughes JR, Foerg F, Badger G. 1993. Achieving cocaine abstinence with a behavioral approach. American Journal of Psychiatry 150:763–769.

Holder HD, Blose JO. 1992. The reduction of health care costs associated with alcoholism treatment: a 14-year longitudinal study. Journal of Studies on Alcohol 53:293–302.

Hubbard RL, Marsden ME, Rachal JV, Harwood HJ, Cavanaugh ER, Ginzburg HM. 1989. Drug Abuse Treatment: A National Study of Effectiveness. Chapel Hill: University of North Carolina Press.

IOM (Institute of Medicine). 1990. Treating Drug Problems. Gerstein DR, Harwood HJ, eds. Washington, DC: National Academy Press.

IOM (Institute of Medicine). 1995. Federal Regulation of Methadone Treatment. Rettig R, Yarmolinsky A, eds. Washington, DC: National Academy Press.

Khalsa HK, Anglin MD. 1991. Treatment effectiveness for cocaine abuse. In: Cocaine Today and Its Effects on the Individual and Society (United Nations Interregional Crime and Research Institute Monograph). 89–98. UNICRI Pub. No. 44.

Kreek MJ. 1992. Rationale for maintenance pharmacotherapy of opiate dependence. In: O'Brien CP, Jaffe JH, eds. Addictive States. New York: Raven Press. 205–230.

Leukefeld CG, Tims FM. 1993. Treatment of cocaine abuse and dependence: directions and recommendations. In: Tims FM, Leukefeld CG, eds. Cocaine Treatment: Research and Clinical Perspectives (NIDA Research Monograph No. 135: 260–266). Rockville, MD: NIDA.

McLellan AT, Arndt IO, Metzger DS, Woody GE, O'Brien CP. 1993. The effects of psychosocial services in substance abuse treatment. Journal of the American Medical Association 269:1953–1959.

McLellan AT, Woody GE, Metzger D, Alterman AI, O'Brien CP. 1994. Is Treatment for Substance Abuse "Worth It?": Public Health Expectations, Policy-Based Comparisons. Presentation at the 20th Anniversary Celebration of NIDA, Bethesda, MD, September 20, 1994.

McLellan AT, Alterman AI, Metzger DS, Grissom GR, Woody GE, Luborsky L, O'Brien CP. In Press. Similarity of outcome predictors in opiate, cocaine and alcohol treatments: role of treatment services. Journal of Clinical and Consulting Psychology.

Means LB, Small M, Capone DM, Capone TJ, Condren R, Peterson M, Hayward B. 1989. Client demographics and outcome in outpatient cocaine treatment. International Journal of Addictions 24:765–783.

NIDA (National Institute on Drug Abuse). 1989. Methadone maintenance: an adequate dose is vital in checking the spread of AIDS. NIDA Notes 4(3):3.

OTA (Office of Technology Assessment). 1990. The Effectiveness of Drug Abuse Treatment: Implications for Controlling AIDS/HIV Infection. Washington, DC: OTA. OTA-BP-H-73. AIDS Related Issues Background Paper 6.

Prendergast ML, Anglin MD, Maugh TH, Hser Y. In press. The Effectiveness of Treatment for Drug Abuse. Draft manuscript prepared April 7, 1994 for NIDA Treatment Services Research Branch. Los Angeles: UCLA Drug Abuse Research Center.

Rawson RA, Obert JL, McCann MJ, Castro FG, Ling W. 1991. Cocaine abuse treatment: a review of current strategies. Journal of Substance Abuse 3:457–491.

Rawson RA, Obert JL, McCann MJ, Ling W. 1993. Neurobehavioral treatment for cocaine dependency: a preliminary evaluation. In: Tims FM, Leukefeld CG, eds. Cocaine Treatment: Research and Clinical Perspectives (NIDA Research Monograph 135:92–115). Rockville, MD: NIDA.

Rydell C, Everingham S. 1994. Controlling Cocaine: Supply Versus Demand Programs. Santa Monica, CA: RAND Drug Policy Research Center. MR-331-ONDCP/A/DPRC.

SAMHSA (Substance Abuse and Mental Health Services Administration). 1994. Client Data System FY 1992: Opiate and Cocaine/Crack Admissions to Treatment. Prepared under contract for the Office of Applied Studies.

Strain EC, Stitzer ML, Liebson IA, Bigelow GE. 1993. Dose-response effects of methadone in the treatment of opiate dependence. Annals of Internal Medicine 119:23–27.

Tims FM, Fletcher BW, Hubbard RL. 1991. Treatment outcomes for drug abuse clients. In: Pickens RW, Leukefeld CG, Schuster CR, eds. Improving Drug Abuse Treatment (NIDA Research Monograph 106:93–113). Rockville, MD: NIDA.

U.S. DHHS (U.S. Department of Health and Human Services). 1993. National Drug and Alcoholism Treatment Unit Survey (NDATUS) 1991 Main Findings Report. DHHS Publication No. (SMA) 93–2007.

Washton AM, 1990. Structured outpatient treatment of alcohol vs. drug-dependencies. Recent Developments in Alcoholism 8:285-304.

Washton AM, Stone-Washton N. 1993. Outpatient treatment of cocaine and crack addiction: a clinical perspective. In: Tims FM, Leukefeld CG, eds. Cocaine Treatment: Research and Clinical Perspectives (NIDA Research Monograph 135:15–30). Rockville, MD: NIDA.

Weisner C, McLellan AT. 1994. Achieving the Public Health Potential of Substance Abuse Treatment: Implications for Patient Referral, Treatment "Matching" and Outcome Evaluation. Presentation at National Institute on Drug Abuse Technical Review: Health Services Research, April 1994.

Wyatt RJ, de Saint Ghislain I. In press. Research as an investment. In: Moscarelli M, Sartorius N, eds. The Economics of Schizophrenia. New York: John Wiley and Sons.

5

Treatment Financing and
Trends in Health Insurance

The financing of treatment is often cited by the pharmaceutical industry as yet another deterrent to the development of anti-addiction medications. Prominent reasons for industry hesitancy are the fact that few patients have private insurance and there is a concomitant need to rely on direct public subsidies to pay for treatment (Chapter 4; IOM Workshop, June 13, 1994).

This chapter examines the financing of treatment in greater depth to uncover the full range of financing disincentives and incentives to the development of anti-addiction medications. It highlights the difficulties companies face in launching a new medication with regard to securing treatment financing as presented by a case study on the financing of levo-alpha-acetylmethadol (LAAM).

The financing of treatment for opiate and cocaine dependencies are described separately in this chapter despite the overlap in the clinical populations (Condelli et al., 1991; Batten et al., 1992). From the perspective of pharmaceutical development, the markets for medications are distinct; for example, the size of the market for cocaine treatment is considered larger because there are more cocaine-dependent than opiate-dependent individuals (Chapter 1); also there is the possibility that a cocaine medication will not be a narcotic and not subject to the panoply of federal and state regulations (Chapters 7 and 8). Narcotic medications for the treatment of narcotic addictions are regulated even more severely under the Controlled Substances Act and state statutes than are other narcotics prescribed for the treatment of pain (Figure 5.1; Chapter 7).

120

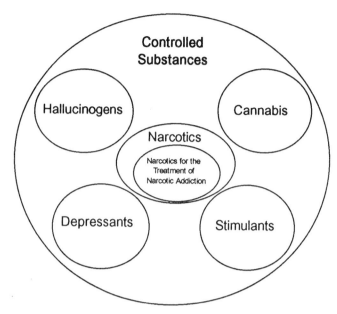

FIGURE 5.1 Narcotics for the treatment of narcotic addiction are a legally-defined subset of narcotics and controlled substances.

FINANCING OF TREATMENT

Financing is generally defined as payment or reimbursement for the cost of treatment made by private insurance, Medicaid, the patients themselves, or other sources. Financing is important to pharmaceutical investment because it has a critical effect on treatment supply and demand for treatment (Rogowski, 1993). Insurance or publicly subsidized coverage increases demand because it improves patients' ability to pay for services. For example, research has shown that people with more generous health insurance buy more prescription drugs and visit doctors more frequently than do those with poorer coverage (Leibowitz et al., 1985; Manning et al., 1988). Likewise, providers who supply treatment tailor facilities and services to maximize their prospects for private, third-party reimbursement or public financing.

The financing of treatment is in a state of transition as a result of the barrage of market forces irrespective, or in anticipation, of future health care reform legislation. A whole new industry of pharmaceutical benefit management, for example, is contributing to immense competitive pressures in the pharmaceutical marketplace for medications to be cost-effective. Benefits also are under increasing scrutiny by insurers who seek to contain costs.

Financing the Treatment of Opiate Addiction

The annual payments for methadone maintenance treatment were estimated at $480 million in fiscal year (FY) 1993. There are an estimated 117,000 patients for whom annual expenditures are about $4,100 each. Those estimates by Harwood and colleagues (1994) are based on extrapolations from the 1991 National Drug and Alcoholism Treatment Survey (NDATUS), which is described in Chapter 4. The vast majority of expenditures are for counseling, medical care, administration, and record keeping. The expenditures for actual medication (methadone or LAAM) are likely to be no more than 10 percent of treatment expenditures, but there is no direct breakdown of treatment financing data to give direct information about the financing of medication as such. Treatment financing data are available only in the aggregate. Despite the lack of available data on the financing of medication, there is information on its retail price. Based on the retail price to clinics, the cost of methadone can be estimated at about $30 million, or about 7 percent of the total cost of treatment (P. Coulis, National Institute on Drug Abuse, personal communication, 1994).

Methadone treatment is financed from a combination of federal, state, local, and private sources. Public sources account for most of the financing, yet there is wide variation from state to state and program to program. The contribution from each of those sources can be estimated from two separate data bases—NDATUS and SADAP, the State Alcohol and Drug Abuse Profile.[1] Financing for methadone treatment falls into 3 categories: public funding, out-of-pocket payments by patients, and private insurance.

Public sources together accounted for $384 million, or about 80 percent of the total payments for methadone treatment in 1993. The federal component, in the form of block grants[2], was about 30 percent of the total. The state component, in the form of direct outlays from the state alcohol and drug agencies, was about 31 percent of the total. The Medicaid component was about 12 percent of the total. The local component, in the form of county or local agency funds, was about 7 percent of the total (Butynski et al., 1994). Medicare plays a negligible

---

[1]SADAP is a voluntary annual survey of funding of publicly supported alcohol and other drug treatment services. With the focus of the survey on programs that receive some state funding, there are virtually no data on private, for-profit programs. SADAP has the advantage of offering trend information because the survey has been collected annually since 1987 by the National Association of State Alcohol and Drug Abuse Directors, Inc. (NASADAD).

[2]The Substance Abuse Prevention and Treatment Block Grant, renamed from the Alcohol, Drug Abuse, and Mental Health Block Grant under the ADAMHA Reorganization Act of 1992 is the source of federal funding.

role primarily because of the younger age and poorer employment history of the drug-dependent population.

Out-of-pocket payments by patients account for 17 percent of the total, or $81.6 million. Private insurance, either in the form of fee-for-service plans or other private plans, such as health maintenance organizations, pays for 2.5 percent of the total, or $12 million. The estimates for the client-paid and private insurance sources are extrapolated from the 1991 NDATUS (H. Harwood, Lewin-VHI, unpublished estimates, 1994).

The financing of methadone treatment is quite different from the financing of other types of medical treatment (Figure 5.2). Public outlays are responsible for 80 percent of payments. Public funding of methadone treatment is far greater than that for all health expenditures, towards which public payments contribute 45.8 percent of the total (CBO, 1993). The composition of the public payers for methadone treatment is quite unusual as most of the public outlays are in the form of direct payments from federal block grants and state alcohol and drug agencies. The only exception is Medicaid which contributes 12 percent of methadone treatment payments, a share similar to Medicaid's contribution of 15.5 percent to all national health expenditures (CBO, 1993).

It is counterintuitive that the Medicaid share is not higher for methadone treatment because many methadone patients are indigent (Chapter 4). There are two reasons for that apparent misperception: first, state Medicaid programs are not required to cover drug abuse treatment, and if they do elect to cover it, the coverage is often limited (GAO, 1991; CRS, 1993b); and second, many drug-dependent patients are ineligible for Medicaid—they meet the low-income criteria, but they do not meet the categorical criteria for Aid to Families with Dependent Children (AFDC) and Supplemental Security Income (SSI).[3] AFDC is targeted to women with dependent children, and SSI is targeted to aged, blind, and disabled persons. Most opiate-dependent persons are young, male, and single (Batten et al., 1992; Price et al., 1991), which usually disqualifies them from AFDC, and they are unlikely to meet the demanding disability criteria for SSI (IOM, 1995). In fact, restrictive Medicaid eligibility is partly responsible for the evolution of the large role for federal block grant and state alcohol and drug agency funding. The ratio of federal block grant to state agency funds for drug abuse treatment (approximately 50:50) is about the ratio of federal to state Medicaid funds in many states, such as New York and California. Thus, the

---

[3]AFDC and SSI are income support programs that confer automatic Medicaid eligibility. At the state's option, Medicaid coverage can be provided for the "medically needy," those individuals who are near poverty but do not qualify as categorically needy because their income is above the mandatory level. For further elaboration on these programs, refer to IOM (1995).

burden of financing of methadone treatment ultimately remains a shared responsibility between the federal and state governments.

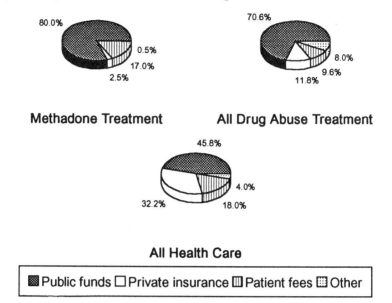

Methadone Treatment   All Drug Abuse Treatment

All Health Care

| ▦ Public funds □ Private insurance ▥ Patient fees ▨ Other |

FIGURE 5.2 Payments for methadone treatment, all types of drug abuse treatment, and all types of health care.
NOTE: Methadone treatment: Total payments, 1993: $480 million. Public funds are divided as follows: federal block grants (30%), state agency (33%), Medicaid (12%), local (5%). Adapted from the 1991 NDATUS by Lewin-VHI. SOURCES: Butynski et al., 1994; Harwood et al., 1994; Lewin-VHI, unpublished estimates, 1994.
All types of drug abuse treatment: Total payments, 1991: $1.2 billion. Public funds are divided as follows: federal (31.4%, including Medicaid, Medicare, and other federal), state and local (39.2%). SOURCE: U.S. DHHS, 1993.
All types of health care: Total payments, 1993: $898 billion. Public funds are divided as follows: Medicaid (15.5%), Medicare (16.8%), other public (13.5%). SOURCE: CBO, 1993.

Federal and state funding has shifted dramatically over the past 20 years. In the 1970s, the federal government had a central role in managing and financing treatment. During the 1980s, the responsibility shifted back to the states, and the federal government created block grants in 1981 to help the states with their new responsibility. In 1987, however, only 15 percent of treatment funding came from block grants. Since then, the block grant contribution has risen substantially, to 30.2 percent, and the state contribution, 45 percent in 1987, has declined to 32.8 percent (Table 5.1). The trends in treatment funding from federal, state, and other sources are mixed. After adjusting for medical inflation, total funding from all sources was greatest in 1976. Thereafter, it declined significantly until 1982, and then began to increase to 1987; the total funding for 1987 was still about 15 percent below that in 1976 (IOM, 1990).

TABLE 5.1 Trends in Financing of State-Supported Alcohol and Other Drug Abuse Services by Largest Funding Sources

Fiscal Year	Federal Block Grant	State Alcohol and Drug Agency	Private Insurance, Client and Patient Fees[1]	Medicaid and Other Public Sources[2]	Total
1987	15%	45%	22%	9%	91%
1988	17%	43%	20%	11%	91%
1989	20%	42%	18%	12%	92%
1990	22.2%	37.8%	15.7%	16.6%	92.3%
1991	29.2%	34.7%	15.5%	13.7%	93.1%
1992	30.2%	32.8%	18.1%	12.3%	93.4%

[1]Also includes court fines. This column renames, but contains the same information as, the SADAP category called "Other Sources."
[2]This column combines the following SADAP categories, "Other State Agency" and "Other Federal Government," in order to capture the federal and state shares of Medicaid, which constitute most of these two categories. There are other state and federal funds included in this column, but they do not come from the federal block grant or from state substance abuse agencies.
NOTE: The percentages in this table do not add up to 100% because this table focuses only on the largest funding sources.

SOURCE: U.S. DHHS, 1987–1992.

Despite the huge public role in financing, the state agencies and the federal government have been unable to exert market leverage to exact manufacturer discounts. Federal block grant funds flow to state alcohol and drug agencies, which administer the funds directly to providers who make pharmaceutical purchases solely for their clinics. Given this funding chain, public agencies do not act the same way that private-sector pharmaceutical benefit managers do when they use collective purchasing strength to negotiate directly with pharmaceutical companies to acquire volume discounts. However, it may well be that pharmaceutical companies even now are deterred from investing because of the perception of potentially strong purchasing power that could be exerted by public agencies in the future.

Private insurance coverage of methadone treatment, at 2.5 percent of the total, is almost insignificant. In contrast, private insurance payments represent 33 percent of all national health expenditures (CRS, 1993a). Upon entering treatment, 5.2 percent of patients list private insurance as the primary source of payment (SAMHSA, 1994). However, because most private policies have restrictions that limit coverage for treatment, most benefits are exhausted after 1 month (Harwood et al., 1994). The group of patients who use insurance (about 11 percent) is largest at private, not-for-profit programs; the greatest percentage of patients paying out-of-pocket (77 percent) is at for-profit facilities (Batten et al., 1992). Patient fees pay for 17 percent of total methadone treatment costs, a share similar to that for all national health expenditures (CBO, 1993). This contradicts the perception that patients are unwilling to pay for treatment.

Financing the Treatment of Cocaine Addiction

There is little data on the financing of treatment specifically for cocaine addiction. NDATUS, the best source, presents data in the aggregate, and with the exception of opiates does not stratify the data by primary drug of abuse. Figure 5.2 provides the most recent published data from 1991 NDATUS on the treatment financing for all drugs of abuse. As stated in Chapter 4, an estimated 30–40 percent of all patients in treatment use cocaine (Batten et al., 1992).

Treatment for cocaine addiction is financed by the same combination of sources as is methadone treatment, but in different proportions. Of the total payments of $1.2 billion for all drug abuse treatment, state and local agencies contributed 39.2 percent, federal block grants contributed 31.4 percent, private insurance contributed 11.8 percent, client and patient fees contributed 9.6 percent, and other sources including private donations and public welfare contributed 8 percent (U.S. DHHS, 1993). Combining all public sources yields a contribution of 70.6 percent, a share that is lower than that for methadone treatment (80 percent, Figure 5.2) but still much higher than that for all health care expenditures (45.8 percent). Similarly, the amount of private insurance payments (11.8 percent) is greater than that for methadone treatment (2.5 percent), but much lower than that for all health care expenditures (33 percent).

FINANCING OF LAAM FOR THE TREATMENT OF OPIATE ADDICTION

LAAM was introduced into clinical practice so recently that its financial profile is somewhat tenuous, mostly because of state financing and regulatory practices. Information in this section is based on interviews with clinic operators, state authorities, and representatives of BioDevelopment Corporation, which manufactures and markets LAAM.

The first sales took place in selected states in April 1994, even though LAAM received Food and Drug Administration (FDA) approval in July 1993. BioDevelopment Corporation officials reports that clinics did not begin to buy the medication any earlier because of state scheduling requirements and state and federal approvals needed for narcotics used in the treatment of narcotic addiction (Chapters 7 and 8). BioDevelopment's monthly revenues since the introduction of LAAM, its only product, began at $3,000 in April and rose to $14,000 by May. Revenues were projected to reach $16,000 by June 1994. Of the 737 dispensing units nationwide[4] already approved by FDA to dispense methadone by June 1994, only 23 had received the separate approval necessary to dispense LAAM.

BioDevelopment set the price for LAAM at about double that for methadone. The average patient can be maintained on LAAM for about $8–$12 for three weekly doses, in comparison with about $5–$8 for seven weekly doses of methadone (irrespective of the number of take-home doses). Some private for-profit clinics in Texas charge LAAM patients an additional $5 per week.

LAAM's higher price is warranted, according to BioDevelopment, for several reasons: first, it is more expensive to manufacture than methadone; second, some patients prefer LAAM because it produces fewer narcotic effects (less sedation, less euphoria); and finally some patients can visit their clinics less often, thereby saving transportation and opportunity costs, because LAAM is administered three times a week. The reduction in dosing frequency is presented as an important advantage to public health, because clinics could increase their patient load. Another advantage promoted by BioDevelopment is that a clinic that uses LAAM exclusively can operate more efficiently because of an estimated 15–20 percent reduction in dispensing and pharmacy services. That is especially important for publicly funded clinics, which generally operate on fixed, sometimes dwindling, budgets. For instance, a clinic that only dispenses LAAM could close on Sunday, when wages are higher. Thus, the higher cost of LAAM relative to methadone might be offset by lower overhead.

State financing has been and is expected to be a major impediment to the sale of LAAM, according to BioDevelopment and clinic operators. State financing practices can be so rigid that they effectively block the introduction and adoption of a new medication. The flow of funds to clinics is dictated by the policies and regulations of two separate state agencies: the state alcohol and drug

---

[4]This figure is the number of dispensing units rather than the number of clinics. FDA licenses dispensing units, and a large clinic with more than one dispensing site, usually on different floors, will be counted more than once. Therefore, this is an overestimate of the number of methadone clinics nationwide (IOM, 1995).

agency, which administers state funds and federal block grants, and the state Medicaid agency, which administers state and federal Medicaid dollars. There is widespread variation in funding practices (IOM, 1995), but either state agency can erect financial barriers to the adoption of a new medication. New York sets a flat daily or weekly fee per patient (which usually includes all services without specifying the amount for medication and dispensing); other states set a flat fee for a "dosing visit," the dispensing of one dose of medication. California authorizes ceilings on the number of publicly funded patients that can be treated at each clinic (Goldstein, 1989). Under these funding practices, LAAM is at a disadvantage because it is more expensive than methadone, the medication for which reimbursement rates have been structured over the past 20 years. To obtain better reimbursement, clinics must petition the appropriate agency for more favorable rates. The alcohol and drug agency in Texas, for example, is not planning to increase reimbursements for LAAM, despite requests from clinic operators (S. Garza, Texas Commission on Alcohol and Drug Abuse, personal communication, 1994). When Medicaid reimbursements fall short, clinics are not generally permitted to bill the patient, and patients are not required to pay the difference.

Financing obstacles are contributing to the stalled market penetration of LAAM. Its higher price might have exacerbated the problem, but the rigidity of the financing structure antedates its introduction. Even one of LAAM's selling points for public health—the prospect of increasing clinic patient loads—has become a disincentive for state alcohol and drug authorities struggling to find additional funding not just for LAAM, but for the higher costs of counseling and comprehensive treatment for possibly more patients. If BioDevelopment Corporation succeeds in securing adequate financing, that will serve as an incentive to other pharmaceutical companies. If not, the future for other opiate medications does not appear encouraging. Therefore, the committee strongly urges state and federal agencies to work together, in the interest of public health and to provide an incentive to pharmaceutical companies, to facilitate the availability of newly approved anti-addiction medications. Possible mechanisms that the states and federal government might consider include requiring all Substance Abuse Block Grant recipients to offer those medications to patients and assuring appropriate financing of new medications by state alcohol and drug agencies and their counterpart Medicaid agencies. Those actions would have the additional benefit of sending a strong signal to the pharmaceutical companies, demonstrating state and federal commitment to the development of anti-addiction medications.

One of the ironies about LAAM's financing is that insured patients, those most likely to afford LAAM, are generally the more stable patients who qualify for the greatest number of methadone take-homes permitted by state and federal regulations (often 6 per week). Those patients appear to have the least incentive to switch to LAAM because they would have to visit the clinic more frequently (M. Parrino, American Methadone Treatment Association, personal communication, 1994) as Federal regulations prohibit LAAM take-home dosing [21 CFR § 291.505(k)(1)(iii)]. In light of the published data, however, that strongly suggests less of an abuse potential with LAAM than methadone (Blaine and Renault, 1976), the committee urges that the FDA and the Drug Enforcement Administration (DEA) reconsider the regulations that prohibit LAAM take-home dosing to permit take-home privileges of LAAM. While the committee realizes that LAAM could be harmful to uninformed, nontolerant, or new patients because of its delayed effect, LAAM take-home privileges could require restrictions similar to methadone take-home privileges. The prohibition on take-homes has been a significant barrier to patient and provider interest in LAAM (Chapter 8).

In conclusion, financing and regulatory obstacles continue to stall the market penetration of LAAM. LAAM's higher price may have exacerbated the problem, but the rigidity of the financing and regulatory structure antedate the introduction of LAAM. If BioDevelopment eventually succeeds in securing adequate financing, that will serve as an incentive to other pharmaceutical companies. If not, the future for other opiate medications does not appear encouraging.

IMPACT OF HEALTH INSURANCE TRENDS ON MEDICATIONS DEVELOPMENT

Changes in health insurance have been occurring in the marketplace long before legislative remedies were proposed. Market-based and legislatively driven reforms, together or in isolation, are important determinants of pharmaceutical investment in the development of medications for opiate or cocaine addiction. The section below presents an analysis of marketplace trends, in an attempt to forecast their effect on pharmaceutical development. In Appendix G, the committee presents an analysis of possible legislative trends in health care reform.

Trends in Drug Abuse Treatment Benefits

There are three related trends in benefits offered under private insurance; an increase in the number of employer health plans that cover drug dependence treatment; a reduction in the coverage for inpatient treatment; and growth in the management of benefits.

Employers have added drug abuse treatment as an employee benefit—either voluntarily or as a result of state law—because of the recognition that dependence on heroin, cocaine, and alcohol reduces worker productivity and contributes to absenteeism, health problems, theft, and accidents. Through annual surveys, the Bureau of Labor Statistics (BLS) has monitored the growth of such benefits. In 1983, benefits were contained in 43 percent of enrollees' medical plans offered by medium and large employers. By 1989, 96 percent offered them (Kronson, 1991). However, across all types of employers, the BLS found greater limitations placed on drug abuse benefits than were placed on other types of medical benefits. Limitations are used to curtail use and to reduce uncertainty about costs to the employer (IOM, 1990). The most common limitations were in the annual number of days of inpatient hospitalization, the number of annual outpatient visits, and separate maximum dollar amounts per year or per lifetime (BLS, 1992). A typical policy restricted inpatient care to 30 days per year, outpatient care to 20 or 30 visits per year, and contained maximum dollar amounts of $25,000 to $50,000 per lifetime for inpatient and outpatient care combined.

The second trend, driven mostly by cost-containment, is a reduction in coverage for inpatient treatment (IOM, 1990). The cost of inpatient drug abuse treatment escalated dramatically during the 1980s, forcing insurers to impose limits on coverage. For example, before the imposition of limits, one study of private insurance claims for about 1 million enrollees (Frank et al., 1991) revealed that inpatient charges per enrollee climbed 32.4 percent between 1986 and 1988, an increase that was almost three times that for all types of medical treatment. After an inpatient limit of 30 days was established, charges increased only 2.2% over a 1-year period. Consistent with this trend, Rawson and co-workers (1991) observed that by the end of the 1980s, cocaine-dependent individuals faced insurance restrictions on the use of hospital-based chemical dependency programs, which often cost $25,000 for a treatment episode. Those programs had been the treatment of choice for those with insurance in the mid-1980s, the peak of the middle-class cocaine epidemic.

Reductions in hospital coverage are more likely to have been felt by cocaine—rather than opiate-dependent patients, because methadone treatment has long been delivered in the outpatient setting. Cocaine-dependent patients who previously sought hospital care in chemical dependency programs are now often treated in 24-hour residential programs. Hospital treatment is typically reserved for drug abuse patients who have concomitant medical and psychiatric problems of a serious nature. According to Rawson and co-workers (1991) the shifting of cocaine-dependent patients to the outpatient setting was motivated principally by the cost concerns of insurers. More recently, Alterman and co-workers (1994) have shown that patients randomly assigned to intensive day hospital treatment for cocaine addiction had as much improvement at less cost than did those assigned to inpatient treatment. The cost of the intensive day hospital (27 hours per week) was only 40–60 percent of inpatient treatment costs (48 hours per week).

Management of benefits, motivated by insurer cost containment policies, attempts to control costs and yield greater efficiency by influencing the treatment decisions of practitioners and patients. Benefits can be managed by a fee-for-service policy through a special carve-out of the drug abuse treatment benefit, through a health maintenance organization (HMO), or through a preferred-provider organization. Benefit management is exerted in a variety of ways, most commonly through preadmission review, case management to refer patients to the most appropriate providers and medically necessary services, and utilization review during and after discharge.

Industry claims of cost containment have begun to be buttressed by academic research. Larson and Horgan (1994) state that managed care can sharply reduce treatment expenditures under private and public health insurance. One of the studies they cite focused on the effect of managed care on 375,000 enrollees in the Massachusetts Medicaid program. Callahan and co-workers (1994) found the initiation of managed care to reduce treatment expenditures per enrollee by 48 percent. Contributing to this overall reduction was a decrease in inpatient expenditures per enrollee of 67 percent and an increase in outpatient expenditures of 8 percent. Overall, the number of patients who received services increased by 5 percent, although this might reflect a higher share of disabled enrollees. There was a 4.6 percent increase in the use of services, primarily as a result of greater usage of methadone services and freestanding detoxification. No direct comparisons of quality of care were possible between managed care and the prior fee-for-service system because of the lack of baseline data. Providers who were surveyed after managed care had been introduced reported a somewhat improved quality of care, and a pilot survey of patients characterized their impressions as "generally positive."

The trend toward expanded benefits should aid pharmaceutical development because of an expected increase in demand for anti-addiction medications. The demand also should increase as a result of the trend in management of benefits, because this approach appears to broaden access to plan members. On balance, the trends in addiction treatment benefits are encouraging.

REFERENCES

Alterman AI, O'Brien CP, McLellan AT, August DS, Snider EC, Droba M, Cornish JW, Hall CP, Raphaelson AH, Schrade FX. 1994. Effectiveness and costs of inpatient versus day hospital cocaine rehabilitation. Journal of Nervous and Mental Disorders 182:157–163.
Batten H, Prottas J, Horgan CM, Simon LJ, Larson MJ, Elliott EA, Marsden ME. 1992. Drug Services Research Survey Final Report: Phase II. Waltham, MA: Bigel Institute for Health Policy, Brandeis University. Contract number 271-90-8319/1. Submitted to the National Institute of Drug Abuse, February 12, 1992.

Blaine JD, Renault PF. 1976. Rx: 3 Times Per Week LAAM Alternative to Methadone. NIDA Research Monograph 8. Rockville, MD: NIDA.

BLS (Bureau of Labor Statistics). 1992. Substance Abuse Provisions in Employee Benefit Plans. Bulletin 2412. Washington, DC: U.S. Department of Labor, BLS.

Butynski W, Reda J, Bartosch W, McMullen H, Nelson S, Anderson R, Ciaccio M, Sheehan K, Fitzgerald C. 1994. State Resources and Services Related to Alcohol and Other Drug Problems for Fiscal Year 1992. Washington, DC: National Association of State Alcohol and Drug Abuse Directors, Inc.

Callahan JJ, Shepard DS, Beinecke RH, Larson M, Cavanaugh D. 1994. Evaluation of the Massachusetts Medicaid Mental Health/Substance Abuse Program. Submitted to the Massachusetts Division of Medical Assistance, Mental Health Substance Abuse Program. Waltham, MA: Institute for Health Policy, Brandeis University.

CBO (Congressional Budget Office). 1993. Estimated Projections of National Health Expenditures, 1993 Update. Washington, DC: CBO.

Condelli WS, Fairbank JA, Dennis ML, Rachal JV. 1991. Cocaine use by clients in methadone programs: significance, scope, and behavioral interventions. Journal of Substance Abuse Treatment 8:203–212.

CRS (Congressional Research Service). 1993a. Medicaid: An Overview. Washington, DC: Library of Congress, CRS. CRS Report No. 93-144 EPW.

CRS (Congressional Research Service). 1993b. Medicaid Services for Substance Abuse Treatment. Washington, DC: Library of Congress, CRS. CRS Report No. 93-764 EPW.

Frank RG, Salkever D, Sharfstein S. 1991. A new look at rising mental health insurance costs. Health Affairs 10:116–23.

GAO (General Accounting Office). 1991. Substance Abuse Treatment: Medicaid Allows Some Services But Generally Limits Coverage. Washington, DC: GAO. HRD 91–92.

Goldstein HM. 1989. The Availability of Methadone Maintenance in California. Drug Abuse Information and Monitoring Project (DAIMP) White Paper Series 9. Los Angeles: UCLA Drug Abuse Research Center, DAIMP. Prepared for the California Department of Alcohol and Drug Programs.

Harwood HJ, Thomsom M, Nesmith T. 1994. Healthcare Reform and Substance Abuse Treatment: The Cost of Financing Under Alternative Approaches. Fairfax, VA: Lewin-VHI.

IOM (Institute of Medicine). 1990. Treating Drug Problems. Gerstein DR and Harwood HJ, eds. Washington, DC: National Academy Press.

IOM (Institute of Medicine). 1995. Federal Regulation of Methadone Treatment. Rettig R, Yarmolinsky A, eds. Washington, DC: National Academy Press.

Kronson ME. 1991. Substance abuse coverage provided by employer medical plans. Monthly Labor Review April:3–10.

Larson M, Horgan CM. 1994. Issues in Calculating the Cost of a Substance Abuse Benefit under Health Care Reform. Presentation at the Legislative Leaders Conference on Substance Abuse Benefits in State Health Care Reform, Denver, CO, May 20–21, 1994. Sponsored by Intergovernmental Health Policy Project.

Leibowitz A, Manning WG, Newhouse JP. 1985. The Demand for Prescription Drugs as a Function of Cost-Sharing. Santa Monica, CA: RAND. RAND/N-2278-HHS.

Manning WG, Newhouse JP, Duan N, Keeler E, Benjamin B, Leibowitz A, Marquis MS, Zwanziger J. 1988. Health Insurance and the Demand for Medical Care: Evidence from a Randomized Experiment. Santa Monica, CA: RAND. RAND Health Insurance Experiment Series RAND/R-3476-HHS.

Price RH, Burke AC, D'Aunno TA, Klingel DM, McCaughrin WC, Rafferty JA, Vaughn TE. 1991. Outpatient drug abuse treatment services, 1988. In: Pickens RW, Leukefeld CG, Schuster CR, eds. Improving Drug Abuse Treatment (NIDA Research Monograph 106: 63–92). Rockville, MD: NIDA.

Rawson RA, Olbert JL, McCann MJ, Castro FG, Ling W. 1991. Cocaine abuse treatment: a review of current strategies. Journal of Substance Abuse 3:457–491.

Rogowski JA. 1993. Private Versus Public Sector Insurance Coverage for Drug Abuse. Santa Monica, CA: RAND Drug Policy Research Center. MR-166-DPRC.

SAMHSA (Substance Abuse and Mental Health Services Administration). 1994. Client Data System FY 1992: Opiate and Cocaine/Crack Admissions to Treatment. Prepared under contract for the Office of Applied Studies.

U.S. DHHS (U.S. Department of Health and Human Services). 1987–1992. State Resources and Services Related to Alcohol and Drug Abuse Problems. Prepared by the National Association of State Alcohol and Drug Abuse Directors, Inc. for the Office of Applied Studies, SAMHSA.

U.S. DHHS (U.S. Department of Health and Human Services). 1993. National Drug and Alcoholism Treatment Unit Survey (NDATUS) 1991 Main Findings Report. DHHS Publication No. (SMA) 93-2007.

6

Training and Education

Pharmaceutical investment in new medications, from discovery to marketing, is expensive and risky (OTA, 1993; Chapter 7), and it depends on a strong infrastructure to support a return on investment. The infrastructure for research and development of a new medication has many components: strong federal leadership and private sector commitment, federal and industry support of research, basic scientists dedicated to elucidating the mechanisms of disease, clinical investigators designing and conducting clinical research and identifying potential leads for new treatments, clinicians specifically trained in the diagnosis and treatment of the disease, health care professionals knowledgeable about recent research findings, adequate reimbursement for treatment, and an educated public that supports effective treatments. In the area of anti-addiction medications development, however, many of those components are scarce or nonexistent.

This chapter explores three paths towards strengthening the clinical research and treatment components of the infrastructure for anti-addiction medications development: increasing the number of clinicians and clinical researchers in the field of addiction research and treatment; providing all physicians with training in the diagnosis and treatment of drug dependence; and expanding the capabilities and coordination of federal drug abuse research centers for all aspects of research, training, treatment, and education.

Drug abuse is a major public health problem in the United States (Chapter 1). The economic consequences of drug abuse are staggering—the United States spends more than $66 billion annually on drug-abuse related health care costs and on the indirect costs of crime, incarceration, and drug supply control (D. Rice, University of California at San Francisco, personal communication). Yet, the federal government has not provided sustained support or innovative programs to increase the number of clinical researchers and clinicians in the field of drug addiction—a critical component of the infrastructure. There are too few clinicians trained in diagnosis and treatment, and there are limited numbers of clinical investigators interested in pursuing careers in drug addiction research. While the biomedical sciences in general are having difficulty in attracting and funding young researchers, especially clinical investigators (IOM, 1988, 1990; NRC, 1994), the numbers being attracted to the field of drug addiction research are particularly sparse. That fact has led addiction medicine to be identified as an orphan field of medicine (IOM Workshop, June 1994).

It is possible, however for the federal government to stimulate the discovery of anti-addiction medications. Historically, there have been other types of medications for which research and development were not initially embraced by the pharmaceutical companies. Comparable to the early history of acquired immune deficiency syndrome (AIDS) research and drug development, for example, the field of addiction treatment is faced with obstacles that include a stigmatized patient population, a lack of specialized clinicians and researchers, and limited scientific knowledge regarding the disease mechanism. Despite those difficulties, federal investment and support in AIDS research has led to an increase in researchers and clinicians and to the development of several medications. During the past 10 years, four medications have been developed and approved for the treatment of AIDS, as compared to three anti-addiction medications in the past 30 years. Given the enormous burden of drug abuse on society, drug abuse research and treatment deserve a similar level of attention and resources from the federal government.

EXPANDING THE CORE OF RESEARCHERS AND CLINICIANS

The critical need for scientists, clinical investigators, and clinicians to specialize in drug addiction research and treatment has been recognized by Congress and the executive branch (ONDCP, 1994; U.S. Congress, 1994). However, there are numerous disincentives to entering this field, such as the perceived low prestige of the field of addiction medicine, low-paying positions, difficulties in conducting clinical research, personal health risks of working with patients who often have serious illnesses (e.g., HIV infection and tuberculosis), uncertain treatment reimbursement, a stigmatized patient population, and the involvement of many patients with crime and the criminal justice system.

Although the limited availability of scientists and clinicians specializing in drug abuse research and treatment has direct consequences for the delivery of health care services and research on new treatments, it has a less obvious, but equally important, effect on pharmaceutical R&D investment. Pharmaceutical companies traditionally market their products to health care professionals and promote their products through personal visits by sales representatives, through journal and mail advertising, and through support of scientific symposia and continuing medical education. Pharmaceutical companies distribute their products through hospital and community pharmacies, pharmacy chains, and distributors. To the extent that the treatment of drug dependence is often delivered outside that system by specialized clinics (e.g., narcotic treatment programs, typically with part-time physicians and limited marketing opportunities for pharmaceutical companies), and to the extent that drug abuse treatment involves many fields of medicine (e.g., family practice, internal medicine, psychiatry), pharmaceutical companies see greater difficulty in marketing anti-addiction medications than in marketing other products. Pharmaceutical firms also rely on academic clinical investigators and practicing clinicians to advise them on drug development issues such as current therapeutic trends, the role of drugs in the overall treatment strategy, unmet medical needs, indications to be evaluated, clinical trial design and appropriate therapeutic endpoints. Therefore, increasing the number of trained specialists is critical to anti-addiction medication development.

Many organizations are involved in efforts to strengthen the infrastructure (Box 6.1), and although some progress has been made, addiction medicine is still a relative unknown to many in the health professions and continues to be neglected by the pharmaceutical industry. Drug abuse treatment is intrinsically interdisciplinary and involves a variety of health care professionals, including counselors, social workers, therapists, psychologists, nurses, and physicians. The committee supports increased training opportunities for all health care profession- als involved in drug abuse treatment, but the focus here is on increasing the numbers of clinical investigators and clinicians working in drug addiction research and treatment.

The following section examines current efforts to increase the numbers of physicians and scientists specializing in drug addiction research and treatment, through the National Institute on Drug Abuse (NIDA) training programs, fellowships offered by private institutions and the government, and certification programs.

Training Programs

The committee heard throughout its work and at its June workshop that there is a severe shortage in the number of clinical investigators in the field of addiction medicine. Physician-researchers are needed to take the lead in developing and implementing clinical research programs on new pharmacological and behavioral treatments. NIDA offers research career development awards to support mentored research by scientists and clinicians interested in pursuing careers as independent investigators. However, there is difficulty in attracting physicians to these programs. The Scientist Development Award for Clinicians (K20) provides drug abuse or mental health research experience for clinically trained individuals, especially physicians; the Scientist Development Award (K21) provides experience for biological or behavioral scientists (NIH, 1993). Stipends for those awards are based on institutional base salaries and range up to $75,000. NIDA funding of research career development awards has increased annually from $507,000 in fiscal year (FY) 1991 (funding five awards) to an FY 1994 estimate of $3.9 million (38 awards) (NIDA, 1994a). However, those programs are not filling the critical shortage of clinical investigators. Only two of the 18 recent applicants for K20 and K21 grants were physicians.

NIDA's $7.9 million training budget for FY 1994 was 2.4 percent of its FY 1994 total extramural research funding. Since FY 1986 NIDA's training budget has averaged 2.0 percent of its extramural research funding (Table 6.1). In contrast, other institutes of the National Institutes of Health (NIH)—and the organization as a whole—have larger proportional training budgets. Since FY 1986 the training budget for the National Institute of Neurological Disorders and Stroke averaged 3.1 percent of total extramural research (2.7 percent in FY 1993), the National Institute on Mental Health averaged 7.7 percent (6.4 percent in FY 1993), and NIH as a whole averaged 4.8 percent (4.3 percent in FY 1993) (NIDA, 1994a). In the FY 1994 bypass budget, NIDA requested an increase in the number of trainees to 440 full-time positions, but only modest increases were funded. For FY 1995 NIDA has requested $17.4 million for research training, which would more than double its training budget (NIDA, 1994b). Actual funding increases are expected to be modest. Funding for the National Research Service Awards (NRSA), the majority of training funding, is appropriated by Congress to NIH as a whole.[1] Once the final appropriation is made, NIDA competes with other NIH institutes for a share of the funds.

Fellowships

Another mechanism for developing expert practitioners, researchers, and teaching faculty is through postresidency fellowships, primarily sponsored by

---

[1]NRSAs fund training opportunities that include predoctoral and postdoctoral research and mentored research for career development. In 1994, NIDA awarded 68 NRSA fellowships (36 predoctoral and 32 postdoctoral) to support individuals working with experienced researchers and 245 NRSA training awards (105 predoctoral and 140 postdoctoral) to support drug abuse research training at public or nonprofit institutions (NIDA, 1994a).

BOX 6.1
Some Organizations Involved in Training and Education

Federal Government
•   National Institute on Drug Abuse (NIDA) supports biomedical and behavioral research, health services research, and research training on drug abuse, including prevention and treatment. NIDA's training opportunities include individual and institutional awards to train predoctoral and postdoctoral clinicians and researchers and support of the Minority Access to Research Careers (MARC) program for minority undergraduate research training. Additionally, NIDA offers mentored research career development programs for scientists and clinicians.

•   Substance Abuse and Mental Health Services Administration (SAMHSA) supports prevention and treatment services for mental health and addictive problems and disorders. The three major components of SAMHSA are the Center for Substance Abuse Treatment (CSAT), the Center for Substance Abuse Prevention (CSAP), and the Center for Mental Health Services (CMHS).
        •   CSAT currently funds 11 addiction training centers that focus on increasing the number and knowledge of health professionals of all disciplines involved in substance abuse treatment. Additionally, CSAT sponsors addiction counselor training programs and develops and disseminates the National HIV/AIDS Training Curriculum.
        •   CSAP has four components in its training system: curriculum development, community prevention training, volunteer training in prevention activities, and the Faculty Development Program, which provides part-time support for faculty in health professional schools to implement or strengthen drug abuse education at their institutions.
        •   CMHS training programs include institutional grants to enhance clinical training of mental health professionals from many disciplines, regional grants for in-service training of practicing mental health professionals, and HIV/AIDS education programs for mental health care providers.

•   Health Resources and Services Administration (HRSA) Bureau of Health Professions has established the Physician Consortium on Substance Abuse Education, which brings together representatives from academia, government agencies, medical professional organizations, and accrediting agencies to focus on drug abuse education for all levels of medical training. Additionally, HRSA has funded faculty development programs in this area.

•   Department of Veterans Affairs (VA) medical centers offer chemical dependency fellowship programs.

Academic Institutions

Individual academic medical centers vary widely in medical school and residency education on drug abuse. Fellowships in addiction medicine are offered at more than 35 institutions, primarily in departments of psychiatry. Health education schools of many disciplines also offer training.

Foundations

Many foundations provide support for drug abuse curriculum development and sponsor educational activities on drug abuse which have included conferences of medical educators, scholarship programs for medical student training on substance abuse, and continuing medical education programs.

Associations and Professional Societies

• **American Academy of Psychiatrists in Alcoholism and Addiction (AAPAA)** has 1,300 members who are board-certified psychiatrists or residents of psychiatry interested in furthering education, research, and treatment of addicted patients. AAPAA offers continuing education review courses and sponsors the publication of *The American Journal on Addictions*.

• **American Society of Addiction Medicine (ASAM)** has a membership of more than 3,000 physicians involved in education, treatment, research and prevention of drug abuse. This organization offers continuing education courses for practicing physicians, administers the independent (non-ABMS) certification in addiction medicine, and sponsors the *Journal of Addictive Diseases*.

• **Association for Medical Education and Research in Substance Abuse (AMERSA)** has a current membership of more than 400 health professional educators. It works to expand drug abuse education and to support faculty and curriculum development. AMERSA was formed in 1976 by many of those involved in the Career Teacher Program. The journal, *Substance Abuse*, is sponsored by AMERSA.

• **College on Problems of Drug Dependence (CPDD)** is an interdisciplinary research society focusing on the problems of drug dependence. Its annual scientific meeting brings together basic scientists and clinical investigators from industry, academia, and government. CPDD sponsors the journal, *Drug and Alcohol Dependence*, which reports scientific research.

• **Professional medical societies** including the Society of Teachers of Family Medicine and the Society of General Internal Medicine offer continuing education courses, develop drug abuse curricula for residency training, and support faculty development efforts.

academic institutions. A 1992–1993 survey conducted by the Center for Medical Fellowships in Alcoholism and Drug Abuse reported 46 fellowship programs inthe addiction field providing 88 fellowship positions, however, only 61 of those positions were filled (Center for Medical Fellowships, 1993). The total number of fellows for 1992–1993, including all training years, was 170. The fellows spent an average of one-third of their time in research, and almost half of their time in patient care. Typically, the fellowship programs are affiliated with psychiatry departments, either solely (85 percent) or jointly with other departments including internal medicine and family practice; few of the programs were affiliated solely with family practice programs or departments.

TABLE 6.1 NIDA Research Training Funding as a Percentage of Total Extramural Research Funding ($ millions)

Year	Research Training						Percent of Total Extramural Research
	Individual		Institutional		Total		
	No.	Amount	No.	Amount	No.	Amount	
1986	24	0.40	48	1.03	72	1.43	2.2
1987	36	0.67	66	1.58	102	1.25	2.0
1988	31	0.57	67	1.73	98	2.30	1.9
1989	35	0.64	52	1.73	87	2.37	1.5
1990	42	0.83	113	2.98	155	3.81	1.4
1991	73	1.26	217	5.55	290	6.81	2.1
1992	61	1.11	224	6.01	285	7.12	2.1
1993	65	1.26	237	6.11	302	7.37	2.2
1994[a]	68	1.38	245	6.52	313	7.90	2.4

[a]Estimate.

SOURCE: NIDA, 1994a.

Fellowships are also offered by NIDA's Addiction Research Center and through the Department of Veterans Affairs. Additionally, NIDA and the Food and Drug Administration (FDA) offer a joint fellowship program aimed at training physicians in drug-abuse treatment research, specifically focused on clinical trials to aid in the development of new anti-addiction medications. That program provides stipends for three clinicians per year to receive 3 years of training through rotations at NIDA's Medications Development Division, the FDA Center for Drug Evaluation and Research, and the NIDA Addiction Research Center. There has been, however, limited applicant response to that program (IOM Workshop, June 1994).

Certification

Board certification has become a "de facto postdoctoral licensing mechanism" for physicians in the United States (Moore and Lang, 1981). Hospitals and managed care companies often require that physicians become board certified in their fields of specialization. In the addiction field, the push for physician certification has resulted in part from third-party insurance carriers' and regulatory agencies' attempts to ascertain the qualifications of physicians responsible for chemical dependency units (Chappel and Lewis, 1992).

The American Board of Medical Specialties (ABMS), a nationally recognized organization with oversight for medical specialty board certification, includes 24 member boards that give annual examinations in core specialties (e.g., internal medicine or psychiatry). Many of these core specialty boards offer certification examinations in subspecialty areas, such as geriatric medicine or addiction psychiatry. In 1991, the American Board of Psychiatry and Neurology (ABPN), an ABMS member board, established the field of addiction psychiatry as a subspecialty. Certification for added qualifications in addiction psychiatry requires ABMS board certification in psychiatry, completion of a fellowship in addiction psychiatry (required after 1998) or extensive clinical practice time with addicted patients, and successful completion of the added qualifications examination (ABPN, 1993).

The American Society of Addiction Medicine offers independent (non-ABMS) certification in addiction medicine for physicians of all specialties. Qualifications for certification include completion of a residency training program, at least one additional year of work in the field of alcohol and drug dependency, and successful completion of the multi-disciplinary certification examination.

The move toward certification is strongly supported by the committee. It increases the number of physicians with a subspecialty in addiction medicine and it increases the knowledge and skills of those physicians who choose certification in addiction medicine.

Conclusions and Recommendations

The committee applauds current efforts aimed at increasing the number of researchers and clinicians in the field of addiction research and medicine, but it recognizes that those efforts have had only limited success. Given the paucity of trained professionals in this area, coupled with other disincentives to the pharmaceutical industry, it is clear that additional measures must be taken to overcome this obstacle.

The committee recommends that the federal government increase its efforts to attract researchers and clinicians to the field of drug addiction treatment. That may be accomplished by implementing one or all of the following options:

•   NIDA's training budget could be increased, but not at the expense of their research programs. Requests from NIDA for large increases in its training budget have not been filled in FY 1993 or FY 1994, and NIDA has received a lower percentage of training funds than several other institutes. Increasing NIDA's training budget such that it will enable NIDA to offer fellowships that are competitive with private sector salaries, and therefore, more attractive to potential candidates would "jump-start" the expansion of the field of drug addiction treatment and research; it could have nationwide impact by increasing the numbers of scientists and physicians recruited, trained, and working in the field of drug addiction.
•   An educational loan repayment program in return for work in drug abuse-related clinical research could attract young physicians with substantial educational debt into careers as clinical investigators.

There is a precedent: the NIH Loan Repayment Program (LRP) for AIDS Research (P.L. 100–607 and P.L. 103–43) allows NIH to repay education loans for NIH scientists, physicians, and registered nurses who spend at least 80 percent of their time involved in AIDS research. Applicants for the LRP program must have qualified educational debt in excess of 20 percent of their annual NIH basic pay or stipend and must be employed under a mechanism that allows for their NIH employment to last a minimum of 2 years (Health Policy and Biomedical Research News of the Week, 1994). To achieve greater national impact, loan repayment for work in the drug addiction field could be extended beyond NIH employees to encompass NIDA trainees and others working in the field.

- Mid-career programs could be developed to encourage a cadre of practicing physicians and scientists to enter the field of drug addiction treatment and research.

Mid-career programs have been sponsored in the field of geriatric medicine with success. The Bureau of Health Professionals and the John A. Hartford Foundation have sponsored one-year training programs for physicians interested in redirecting their careers toward geriatric medicine (IOM, 1993; Robbins, 1993). Similar programs could fill the current needs for physicians in drug addiction treatment and research, while new researchers and physicians are receiving training. In addition, short-term, mid-career training programs should be made available at NIDA's existing research centers and proposed comprehensive drug abuse centers.

INCREASING KNOWLEDGE AND SKILLS AMONG PRIMARY CARE PHYSICIANS

Just as critical as infusing the addiction field with researchers and medical specialists is expanding primary care physicians' knowledge and skills in the diagnosis and treatment of drug abuse. Given the consequences of managed care, health care reform efforts, and the potential for new medications to treat drug addiction, primary care physicians must be able to diagnose drug addiction, and they must be familiar with its treatment modalities. It has been shown that physicians do not diagnose drug abuse disorders with the same accuracy as other chronic diseases (Coulehan et al., 1987; Gopalan et al., 1992). Although they are often the first to see drug-dependent patients (Kamerow et al., 1986). Because of their minimal training in drug abuse, many physicians lack confidence in their diagnostic ability and they are ambivalent or pessimistic about the effectiveness of treatment (Chappel et al., 1977; Cotter and Callahan, 1987). This is not surprising; the curriculum on drug abuse and its treatment varies greatly in medical schools. Over the past 20 years, drug abuse education (most often combining information about alcohol dependence and other addictions) has evolved slowly and has only recently begun to make inroads into the medical school curriculum, residency training programs, and the certification process.

A concerted effort to stimulate medical school education in addiction medicine began in 1972 with the Career Teacher program sponsored by the National Institute on Alcohol Abuse and Alcoholism (NIAAA) and NIDA. Funded in 59 U.S. medical schools, the program trained faculty to develop and implement curricula. That program provided two key elements for raising awareness and expanding knowledge regarding the addiction field—a dedicated faculty member serving as a role model for students and a high profile in medical schools for drug abuse education. During its 10-year existence (1972–1981) the program resulted in an increase in curriculum hours, although the percentage of total time required for drug abuse education remained under 1 percent (Pokorny and Solomon, 1983). Currently, the Center for Substance Abuse Prevention (CSAP) sponsors the Faculty Development Program, begun in 1989, which funds grants to 34 schools of medicine, nursing, social work, and psychology. Each grant provides part-time support for a program director, an evaluator, and three to five faculty fellows with the goal of developing a cadre of faculty to provide leadership in expanding and improving clinical teaching about drug abuse (CSAP, 1994; Fleming et al., 1994a). Faculty development in drug abuse education also has interested medical professional organizations, including the Society of General Internal Medicine and the Society of Teachers of Family Medicine, which, with funding from the Health Resources and Services Administration (HRSA) have developed and implemented faculty development courses (Fleming et al., 1994a).

Additional efforts have been made to define and promote education for primary care physicians. The 1985 Conference on Alcohol, Drugs, and Primary Care Physician Education produced a consensus statement identifying core skills and competencies for primary care physicians and set out educational strategies for implementation (U.S. DHHS, 1985; Lewis et al., 1987). In 1989, under the auspices of the HRSA Bureau of Health Professions, the Physician Consortium on Substance Abuse Education was formed and subsequently drafted recommendations for improving drug abuse education at all levels of medical education (U.S. DHHS, 1991). Work is ongoing to implement those recommendations.

Through private and public funding, model undergraduate medical curricula on alcohol and drug abuse have been developed at several universities. Project ADEPT (Alcohol and Drug Education for Physician Training), a core curriculum, was developed at Brown University, and is used in more than 75 percent of U.S. medical schools (Chappel and Lewis, 1992). Gains have been made in increasing medical school and residency education on drug abuse issues, although it is often fragmented between departments and frequently is not linked to adequate clinical training (Cotter and Callahan, 1987; Lewis et al., 1987). Little attention is being given to cross-cultural and special-population issues in drug abuse education at all levels (U.S. DHHS, 1991).

Required Education in Medical Schools

A 1991–1992 survey of medical schools found that 93 percent of the 124 medical schools responding had at least one curriculum unit in drug abuse; at least two-thirds of those units were required (Fleming et al., 1994b). That was double the amount found in a similar 1986–1987 survey (Davis et al., 1988). The curriculum units ranged from single lectures to clinical experience. The number of departments reporting drug abuse curriculum units ranged by specialty—95 percent of psychiatry, 87 percent of family medicine, 59 percent of pediatrics, 47 percent of internal medicine, 46 percent of emergency medicine, and 45 percent of obstetrics-gynecology departments had at least one unit (Fleming et al., 1994b). The multifaceted nature of the consequences and treatment of drug abuse suggests that medical school education in this field should be cross-departmental and that the basic science and clinical aspects should be sequenced appropriately throughout medical training (Cotter and Callahan, 1987; Burger and Spickard, 1991).

Only eight medical schools surveyed by the Liaison Committee on Medical Education in 1991–1992 had a separate required course on drug abuse (Fleming et al., 1994b). Far more had separate required courses in other special multidisciplinary topics. For example, 17 require a geriatrics course, 32 require a community health course, and 40 require a nutrition course (Fleming et al., 1994b). Few medical schools require clinical experience with drug-abuse patients, and if it is available the clinical experience is often limited to hospital inpatient settings where it is reported that the students are less likely to see the continuum of problems or the range of treatments (Kamerow et al., 1986; Lewis et al., 1987).

Residency Training

Residency education in addiction medicine is highly concentrated in psychiatric programs. A 1991–1992 survey of residency programs in four specialties found that 95 percent of psychiatry programs offered at least one addiction medicine curriculum unit, followed by family medicine (85 percent), pediatrics (59 percent), and internal medicine (47 percent) (Fleming et al., 1994b). Most of the required units were lectures and seminars; the electives were usually 2- to 8-week clinical rotations. Residency programs also rely on inpatient treatment settings for clinical training although most offer clinical exposure to two or more treatment settings (Davis et al., 1988).

The Josiah Macy, Jr. Foundation targeted residency education on drug abuse as the topic for its October 1994 conference. Leadership of the primary care certifying boards and of the residency review committees in internal medicine, family practice, pediatrics, and OBGYN along with business purchasers of health care, state legislative leaders, and drug abuse experts met and reached consensus on the urgency and necessity for primary care residency review committees to require drug abuse education for all residents under their supervision. Additionally, consensus was reached on the need for certifying boards to better reflect in their evaluation process the clinical magnitude of the drug abuse problem (D.

Lewis, Brown University, personal communication).

Continuing Education

Most currently practicing physicians had received minimal formal training—if any—in the diagnosis or treatment of drug abuse while they were in medical school or during their residencies. Continuing medical education (CME) can fill the gap, and several organizations, including the American Society of Addiction Medicine and the American Society for Medical Education and Research in Substance Abuse conduct workshops and conferences that prepare faculty for teaching continuing medical education courses. National professional organizations and state medical societies are also key to CME efforts. For example, the American Medical Association, the American College of Physicians, the Society of Teachers of Family Medicine, the Ambulatory Pediatric Association, and the American College of Obstetrics and Gynecology have all prepared continuing education materials, workshops, and courses in this field. The transfer of new research findings on treatment is especially critical as greater numbers of primary care physicians become involved in diagnosing and treating drug-dependent patients.

Conclusions and Recommendations

Increasing the depth and breadth of drug abuse education at all levels of physician training will result in heightened awareness of the physiological, psychological, and behavioral components of addiction and heightened understanding of the effectiveness of and the need for a range of treatment modalities. By understanding the spectrum and effectiveness of treatment services, physicians will be able to recommend the most appropriate and cost-effective intervention for the individual patient (Simek-Downing and Forman, 1987).

The committee recommends an increased emphasis on drug abuse education throughout medical school and primary care residency programs. To accomplish this, the following could be implemented:

•   Drug abuse education could follow a systematic, integrated approach to coordinate the curriculum across specialty departments.

• Training institutions could develop affiliations with community-based treatment centers, where feasible, to provide student access to multiple treatment settings.

• The National Board of Medical Examiners[2] and the primary care specialty boards of the American Board of Medical Specialties (ABMS) could pay increased attention to drug abuse issues, skills, and knowledge on their examinations for certification.

• Faculty development programs could receive increased federal support. CSAP's Faculty Development Program which trains medical school faculty members to serve as role models, educators, and mentors in the field of drug abuse research and treatment, is a good model.

COMPREHENSIVE DRUG ABUSE CENTERS

The goal of a solid infrastructure needed to support anti-addiction medications development and comprised of specialists and primary care physicians who are knowledgeable in the diagnosis and treatment of drug abuse, can be realized in part through the implementation of comprehensive, multidisciplinary drug abuse centers recommended by the committee (Chapter 2). The centers of excellence would focus on all aspects of research and treatment, and they would offer the added benefit of serving as training sites for new investigators and mid-career physicians entering the field. They also would be clinical training sites for medical students and residents as they learn to diagnose and treat drug-dependent patients. A characterization of the centers, as envisioned by the committee, is provided below. Additionally, current NIDA and Substance and Mental Health Services Administration (SAMHSA) centers are briefly described and options for implementation of the centers are given.

Proposed Model

For optimal effectiveness the centers should have clinical research, treatment, basic research, and training components. Built around a core clinical research program with both inpatient and outpatient treatment capability, they could be funded directly using the model of the National Cancer Institute's (NCI) Comprehensive Cancer Centers (Box 6.2), as discussed in Chapter 2.

---

[2]The National Board of Medical Examiners prepares and administers to medical students a two-part examination that is accepted by individual states as part of licensing.

BOX 6.2
NCI Cancer Centers Program

Begun in the early 1960s, NCI currently supports 55 research centers with diverse focus, structure, size, and funding.

•   **Basic science cancer centers** are primarily engaged in basic laboratory research.
•   **Clinical cancer centers** focus on basic and clinical research.
•   **Comprehensive cancer centers** are multidisciplinary and are designated as meeting NCI's criteria for strong basic and clinical research programs, state-of-the-art patient care, strong participation in NCI-designated high-priority clinical trials, significant prevention and control research, and community outreach activities.
•   **Consortium centers** focus on cancer control and prevention research and work with state and local public health agencies.

The centers are funded through a variety of sources, including the cancer center core grants (P-30 grants from NCI), which cover centralized administrative and program costs including personnel, shared resources, and services (including laboratory equipment), development, planning, and evaluation.

SOURCES: IOM, 1989; NCI, 1993.

The core clinical research program would not be linked to any given research project but would be available to investigators for specific projects and used as a site for training. Pilot projects could be reviewed by a local committee that would decide which proposals could make use of the core treatment unit for research. It would be expected that many of these pilot projects would result in peer-reviewed research project grant (R01) funding. The core treatment unit of the comprehensive center would provide state-of-the-art patient care, serving as a valuable community treatment resource—treatment costs could be supported in part by community or state block grant funding administered by the Center for Substance Abuse Treatment (CSAT). Strong participation in NIDA- and NIH-designated high-priority clinical trials and sponsorship of community outreach activities would be additional priorities for the centers.

An equally essential component of the comprehensive center would be the conduct of preclinical research and the timely transfer of basic research findings to the clinical arena, which should result in the incorporation of pertinent information into clinical protocols to improve their viability. Collaboration between preclinical and clinical researchers is essential and at a minimum should involve regular interdisciplinary seminars that would be expected to lead to collaborative projects.

The training component of the comprehensive centers should involve undergraduates and graduate students, to train physicians and other health care professionals including social workers, nurses, psychologists, and rehabilitation counselors. The center training programs also should include a postdoctoral training program primarily for research, but including training in treatment techniques. Training programs should include funding for faculty and administrative support of training. Competitive salaries for trainees are essential, given the precarious financial situations of most recent medical graduates, and a loan forgiveness program should be explored for trainees in the centers.

The comprehensive centers should be encouraged to develop collaborative ties with the pharmaceutical industry. This would involve testing new medications in preclinical laboratories and conducting clinical trials in the core treatment units. By supplying clinical trial site capability, the centers would provide industry with an incentive to develop anti-addiction medications. The centers would screen patients and obtain the necessary regulatory approvals—overcoming many of the hurdles cited by industry as strong disincentives.

Existing Research and Training Centers

To expand on its recommendation (Chapter 2), the committee explored the existing research and training centers sponsored by NIDA and SAMHSA.

CSAT Centers

The Center for Substance Abuse Treatment initiated its addiction training center (ATC) program in FY 1993 to link publicly funded addiction treatment and recovery programs with institutions that train health and allied health practitioners. The centers serve as training sites for students, provide continuing education to currently practicing treatment staff, and strengthen the drug abuse curriculum within the participating institutions. All ATCs are multidisciplinary and provide training opportunities for addiction counselors and other professionals, including social workers, marriage and family therapists, psychologists, psychiatrists, and primary care physicians and nurses. ATC funds are used to develop clinical training programs, support faculty, and conduct training needs assessments.

Implementation of the program began in FY 1994, and 11 centers are now funded through cooperative agreements—three through state alcohol and other drug addiction agencies, and eight at academic institutions (including three medical-school based-programs).

NIDA Research Centers

In FY 1993 NIDA funded 23 specialized research centers through the P50 Specialized Center extramural grant mechanism, at a cost of $24 million. Specialized centers are multiple-investigator, long-term programs planned around a major research objective or theme. Funded centers cover all aspects of NIDA's mission. Additionally, NIDA has funded treatment research units (TRUs), which conduct clinical studies examining multiple aspects of treatment. Initially funded as research demonstration grants, TRUs now apply competitively for new center grants as they come up for renewal. NIDA's intramural research center, the Addiction Research Center in Baltimore, Maryland, is the site for clinical and basic research on behavioral and pharmacological treatments.

The FY 1995 Department of Health and Human Services appropriations bill calls on NIDA to "support up to five multidisciplinary comprehensive substance abuse centers that will undertake research, service, and training activities to demonstrate the effectiveness of such coordinated activities focused on women, children, and minorities" (U.S. Congress, Senate, 1994). The committee supports the implementation of those centers and stresses the importance of a multidisciplinary effort.

Conclusions and Recommendations

Upon examination of the CSAT and NIDA centers, it appears that there is an opportunity for collaboration. Many of the individual components necessary for the centers, as recommended by the committee, are currently in place. A coordination of efforts between NIDA and SAMHSA could increase the number of facilities available to patients, increase services, enhance research opportunities, and provide additional training opportunities without the need for a concomitant increase in funding. A possible NIDA/SAMHSA collaboration effort could be the use of the ATCs as sites for treatment or prevention research. The committee envisions the comprehensive centers as maximizing effective research and implementing innovative and effective drug abuse treatments.

The committee recommends that comprehensive drug abuse centers be developed to engage in and coordinate all aspects of drug-abuse research, treatment, and education. Further, the committee recommends that NIDA and SAMHSA work together to coordinate

the effective and efficient use of existing centers by adding, where feasible, research, training, and/or treatment components.

The enormous public health and societal costs of drug abuse justify federal funding of comprehensive centers that will train physicians and scientists, provide state-of-the-art treatment, and expand basic research. The committee is aware of federal budgetary constraints and has therefore recommended a mechanism of cooperation between existing resources and capabilities, by expanding the mission and goals of existing NIDA and SAMHSA centers.

SUMMARY

The current involvement of the research and medical communities in research on and treatment for drug abuse is limited. Few clinicians and clinical researchers have been interested in pursuing careers in drug abuse research and treatment, and current efforts, through fellowships, traineeships, research development awards, and certification, have not attracted sufficient interest in the drug addiction field. This shortage of medical specialists has had a negative effect on the pharmaceutical industry.

All physicians need to be educated in diagnosing and treating the chronic nature of drug abuse. Current efforts must be strengthened to increase medical school and primary care residency curricula, provide faculty development programs, and expand continuing medical education.

Comprehensive drug abuse centers, as recommended by the committee, could fulfill the multiple goals of providing sites for state-of-the-art drug abuse treatment and research while serving as training facilities for generalists and specialists.

As the societal costs of drug abuse increase, it is time to address the shortage of specialists and the inadequacy of drug abuse education. Those efforts will strengthen the infrastructure needed for research and treatment and will encourage pharmaceutical investment in this field.

REFERENCES

ABPN (American Board of Psychiatry and Neurology). 1993. Information for Applicants for Added Qualifications. Deerfield, IL:ABPN.

Burger MC, Spickard WA. 1991. Integrating substance abuse education in the medical school curriculum. American Journal of the Medical Sciences 302:181–184.

Center for Medical Fellowships in Alcoholism and Drug Abuse. 1993. Postgraduate Medical Fellowships in Alcoholism and Drug Abuse. New York: New York University School of Medicine, Department of Psychiatry.

Chappel JN, Jordan RD, Treadway BJ, Miller PR. 1977. Substance abuse attitude changes in medical students. American Journal of Psychiatry 134:379–384.

Chappel JN, Lewis DC. 1992. Medical education in substance abuse. In: Lowinson JH, Ruiz P, Millman RB, eds. Substance Abuse: A Comprehensive Textbook. 2nd ed. Baltimore: Williams & Wilkins. 958–969.

Cotter F, Callahan C. 1987. Training primary care physicians to identify and treat substance abuse. Alcohol Health and Research World, Summer:70–73.

Coulehan JL, Zettler-Segal M, Block M, McClelland M, Schulberg HC. 1987. Recognition of alcoholism and substance abuse in primary care patients. Archives of Internal Medicine 147:349–352.

CSAP (Center for Substance Abuse Prevention). 1994. CSAP Training System: Faculty Development Program Information Sheet.

Davis AK, Cotter F, Czechowicz D. 1988. Substance abuse units taught by four specialties in medical schools and residency programs. Journal of Medical Education 63:739–746.

Fleming M, Barry K, Davis A, Kahn R, Rivo M. 1994a. Faculty development in addiction medicine: Project SAEFP, a one-year follow-up study. Educational Research and Methods 26:221–225.

Fleming M, Barry K, Davis A, Kropp S, Kahn R, Rivo M. 1994b. Medical education about substance abuse: changes in curriculum and faculty between 1976 and 1992. Academic Medicine 69:362–369.

Gopalan R, Santora P, Stokes EJ, Moore RD, Levine DM. 1992. Evaluation of a model curriculum on substance abuse at the Johns Hopkins University School of Medicine. Academic Medicine 67:260–266.

Health Policy and Biomedical Research News of the Week ("The Blue Sheet"). 1994. NIH Loan Repayment Program for AIDS Research. 37(28):S4. July 13, 1994.

IOM (Institute of Medicine). 1988. Resources for Clinical Investigation. Washington, DC: National Academy Press.

IOM (Institute of Medicine). 1989. A Stronger Cancer Centers Program. Washington, DC: National Academy Press.

IOM (Institute of Medicine). 1990. Funding Health Sciences Research: A Strategy to Restore Balance. Washington, DC: National Academy Press.

IOM (Institute of Medicine). 1993. Strengthening Funding in Geriatrics for Physicians. Washington, DC: National Academy Press.

Kamerow DB, Pincus HA, MacDonald DI. 1986. Alcohol abuse, other drug abuse, and mental disorders in medical practice. Journal of the American Medical Association 255:2054–2057.

Lewis DC, Niven RG, Czechowicz D, Trumble JG. 1987. A review of medical education in alcohol and other drug abuse. Journal of the American Medical Association 257:2945–2948.

Moore FD, Lang SM. 1981. Board-certified physicians in the United States. New England Journal of Medicine 304:1078–1084.

NCI (National Cancer Institute). 1993. Cancer Facts: The National Cancer Institute Cancer Centers Program. July 1993.

NIDA (National Institute on Drug Abuse). 1994a. Research Training Trends FY1994. Rockville, MD: NIDA Office of Science Policy, Education and Legislation.

NIDA (National Institute on Drug Abuse). 1994b. National Institute on Drug Abuse 1995 Budget Estimate. Rockville, MD:NIDA.

NIH (National Institutes of Health), Division of Research Grants. 1993. The K Awards. Bethesda, MD:NIH.

NRC (National Research Council), Commission on Life Sciences. 1994. The Funding of Young Investigators in the Biological and Biomedical Sciences. Washington, DC: National Academy Press.

ONDCP (Office of National Drug Control Policy). 1994. National Drug Control Strategy: Reclaiming Our Communities from Drugs and Violence. Washington, DC: Executive Office of the President, ONDCP.

OTA (Office of Technology Assessment). 1993. Pharmaceutical R&D: Costs, Risks, and Rewards. Washington, DC: U.S. Government Printing Office. OTA-H-522.

Pokorny AD, Solomon J. 1983. A follow-up survey of drug abuse and alcoholism teaching in medical schools. Journal of Medical Education 58:316–321.

Robbins LJ. 1993. Mid-career faculty development awards in geriatrics: does retraining work? Journal of the American Geriatrics Society 41:570–571.

Simek-Downing L, Forman SI. 1987. The teaching of substance abuse: a national survey and a residency training curriculum. Substance Abuse 8:42–52.

U.S. Congress, Senate. 1994. Departments of Labor, Health, and Human Services, and Education and Related Agencies Appropriation Bill, 1995. 103d Cong., 2d sess. S. Report 103–318.

U.S. DHHS (U.S. Department of Health and Human Services). 1985. Consensus Statements from the Conference Alcohol, Drugs, and Primary Care Physician Education: Issues, Roles, Responsibilities. November 12–15, 1985.

U.S. DHHS (U.S. Department of Health and Human Services). 1991. Policy Report of the Physician Consortium on Substance Abuse Education. Washington, DC: U.S. Government Printing Office. Publication No. HRSA-P-DM-91-3.

7

Federal Laws and Regulations

This chapter and the next discuss the issue of federal and state laws and regulations and the disincentives in developing new anti-addiction medications to the industry. This chapter includes a discussion of the drug-development process, focusing on the multiple interactions between the private sector and federal regulatory agencies, specifically the Food and Drug Administration (FDA) and the Drug Enforcement Administration (DEA), necessary to develop and bring to market an approved anti-addiction medication. This chapter also presents recommendations aimed at accelerating drug discovery and development by removing obstacles to the private sector.

CREATION OF A DRUG BY THE
PHARMACEUTICAL INDUSTRY

More than 90 percent of new drugs are discovered by scientists in the pharmaceutical industry (Kaitin et al., 1993; PMA, 1993b). With rare exceptions, the remainder are derived from the work of academic or government scientists (Kaitin et al., 1993). Even for drugs discovered outside the industry, a partnership or licensing agreement with a drug firm is ultimately necessary for development, manufacturing, and marketing. The process used by the pharmaceutical industry to turn a compound into an agent that can be used by patients (e.g., a tablet or an injectable medicine) can be divided into three stages (Figure 7.1): discovery, development, and marketing (Knoop and Worden, 1988; Spilker and Cuatrecasas, 1990; Agersborg, 1993).

Drug discovery consists of a complex set of laboratory research activities, conducted mainly by chemists and pharmacologists (or molecular biologists in the case of the biotechnology industry), from which emerges a compound or a set of related compounds with a specified biological activity, e.g., inhibition of a key enzyme or receptor. The hope is that such a compound, when subjected to further testing (the process called *drug development*), will prove to be a useful therapeutic agent for a disease in which, e.g., that enzyme or receptor plays a role. New compounds are identified through such approaches as screening large numbers of compounds for the desired biological activity, optimizing molecular structures, using computer-assisted molecular modeling, and testing active compounds in animal models of the relevant disease, when such models exist (Spilker and Cuatrecasas, 1990; PMA, 1993a; Rapaka and Hawks, 1993).

Scientists engaged in drug discovery use the scientific techniques of basic biomedical research, but the goals of the enterprises are different. The purpose of basic research is to advance knowledge and to make it available to the scientific community at large. Basic research is usually funded by government and conducted by academic or government scientists, and its product is public information in written, visual or electronic form. In contrast, the purpose of drug discovery is to identify new substances of potential value in the treatment or prevention of disease. Drug discovery makes use of basic biomedical knowledge, but its end products are a new chemical entity and information on what it does; much of this information is considered proprietary, and new chemical entities are patentable as inventions. Drug discovery as an organized enterprise takes place almost exclusively in the pharmaceutical industry. When a new drug is discovered outside the pharmaceutical industry, it is usually a biotechnology product that is an outgrowth of basic research (an event that is likely to become more common) or a product of a collaborative government-industry or university-industry partnership.

Drug development consists of studies on a potential new drug to determine what it does in humans, whether it is safe and effective for the treatment or prevention of a disease, and whether it is properly labeled. The studies include toxicity studies in animals and clinical studies in humans that are customarily divided into three phases:

- *Phase I* clinical trials in which healthy volunteers receive the drug, and tests are conducted to determine pharmacological information including absorption, blood concentrations, metabolism, initial side effects and, if possible, mechanism of action and efficacy.
- *Phase II* clinical trials involve several hundred patients in which evidence on efficacy and dose-response relationships are obtained.

- *Phase III* clinical trials involve several hundred to several thousand patients in which efficacy and safety are demonstrated in hospital and outpatient settings.

During drug development, the formulations to be marketed (e.g., tablets, capsules, injections) are also developed, and the manufacturing process is scaled up progressively and optimized (Figure 7.1) (Spilker and Cuatrecasas, 1990).

When a compound is ready for the first clinical study in humans (Phase I), it falls under the regulatory authority of FDA and an investigational new drug (IND) application is submitted to the agency. During the remainder of the drug-development period, there is extensive interaction with FDA that includes consultation on the development plan and protocols, the submission of data on serious and unexpected adverse events, and the submission of periodic reports. When the manufacturer has completed the drug-development program, all the information on the formulations, the manufacturing process and plant, toxicity in animals, and clinical effects in humans is submitted in a new drug application (NDA). An important document in the NDA is the proposed package insert, which states that the drug has been shown to be safe and effective and provides directions for use. The NDA is then reviewed by FDA, often with considerable interaction between the agency and the manufacturer; the process might include open review by an advisory committee. If all parts of the NDA are judged to meet the standards prescribed by federal law and regulations, it is approved.

The final step in the creation of a new drug is *marketing*. This ordinarily lasts many years unless (as happens rarely) the drug must be withdrawn because of a safety problem. An important characteristic of the marketing period, not widely recog.nized by the public, is that new uses for a drug are often found after initial marketing as the result of serendipitous discovery by an astute clinician or planned studies by clinical investigators in new patient populations. Sometimes such a new use is more important medically than the use for which the drug was originally developed. The discovery of new uses after initial marketing has proved to be a particularly powerful route to innovation for psychoactive drugs, inasmuch as their effects are not easily predicted from animal models and must usually be identified and proved in humans. Indeed, most of the drugs now in use or in the later stages of evaluation by NIDA for the treatment of opiate or cocaine addiction were originally developed for other medical indications (Wesson and Ling, 1991; NIDA, 1990).

The total cost of creating (discovering, developing, and marketing) a new drug has been analyzed in several studies (Wiggins, 1987; Grabowski and Vernon, 1990; DiMasi et al., 1991) and recently reviewed by the Office of Technology Assessment (OTA, 1993). OTA concluded that "in 1990 dollars, the mean cash outlay required to bring a new drug to market (including the costs of failures along the way) was approximately $127 million for drugs first entering human testing in the 1970s." If capitalized costs (the so-called "cost of time") and tax deductions are considered, the after-tax cost per marketed drug estimated by OTA was "somewhere between $140 and $194 million (in 1990 dollars)." A little more than half the total cost went to preclinical activities—such as drug discovery, chemical synthesis, formulation development, and toxicology—and the remainder went to clinical development. The mean time to create a successful drug was about 12 years. Corresponding figures for the biotechnology industry are not available.

To assess the adequacy of the budget of the NIDA Medications Development Division (MDD), it is most useful to consider actual cash outlays by pharmaceutical companies, inasmuch as the capitalizing of expenditures and tax deductions do not apply to MDD. In this context, the cash outlay for Phase III studies of marketed drugs was estimated by DiMasi and co-workers (1991) to be $14.3 million in 1990 dollars; that figure was supported by OTA (1993). Those costs reportedly rose rapidly—faster than the rate of general inflation—during the 1980s and presumably continue to do so.

On the basis of those figures and informal estimates given by the pharmaceutical executives who met with the committee, the committee believes that $10–40 million is a reasonable estimate for the average cash outlay to develop a major new indication for an already-approved drug. The cash outlay for the full development of a new compound would presumably be near the industry average, i.e., in the range of $100–200 million. For a shared development program—MDD in partnership with a private organization—in which the government supported clinical development, the cash outlay of public funds would be about half the total cost.

Individual pharmaceutical and biotechnology companies have continuing research programs searching for new psychoactive chemicals; some might also have marketed drugs that could be useful in treating one aspect or another of addiction in addition to their primary uses. Individual firms also have the technology for developing, manufacturing, and marketing such drugs. NIDA has research funds to support the development of improved animal models and screening techniques, an operating clinical investigator network, funds to support the clinical development of new drugs and new indications, and a relationship of trust with FDA. Given the enormous amounts of time and money required for pharmaceutical research and development, a collaborative approach between the government and the private sector that pulls complementary resources together appears to be highly desirable.

Chapter 3, in its assessment of MDD, considered the interactions between the private sector and NIDA. The remainder of this chapter addresses the ways in which FDA and DEA interact with the private sector and provides committee recommendations to remove federal regulatory disincentives.

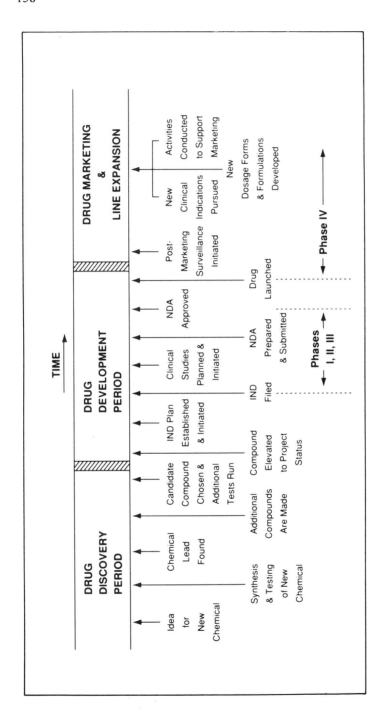

Figure 7.1 Pipeline concept of drug development. Some major activities that occur during discovery, development, and marketing are illustrated on the timeline. Modified with permission from Raven Press. SOURCE: Spilker, 1989.

FOOD AND DRUG ADMINISTRATION

Complaints that the traditional FDA drug-approval process is too slow and discourages drug development are not new. In recent years, however, the traditional process has undergone changes designed to expedite FDA review and to expand the use of experimental treatments under some circumstances. The User Fee Law was passed in 1991 to expedite review and approval of new drugs. In addition, the federal Food, Drug, and Cosmetic Act (FDCA) provides special incentives to manufacturers of particular categories of drugs. These incentives—such as accelerated approval, treatment INDs, and orphan exclusivity—are also available to manufacturers of new anti-addiction drugs. For example, LAAM (levo-alpha-acetylmethadol), which on July 9, 1993, became the first narcotic maintenance drug approved since methadone, was granted orphan exclusivity for use in the treatment of heroin addiction suitable for maintenance with opiate agonists. LAAM also was given an expedited final review by FDA (see LAAM case study in Chapter 8).

The recent changes to the traditional drug-approval process might provide additional opportunities for encouraging and expediting the development of anti-addiction medications.

Recent Initiatives to Expedite Availability of New Drugs

Of particular importance is a series of initiatives intended to expedite the availability of drugs to treat serious and life-threatening diseases for which no adequate therapeutic alternatives exist. The acquired immune deficiency syndrome (AIDS) crisis was the driving force behind these efforts, but products intended to treat a variety of other conditions—including drug addiction—properly qualify for treatment under these initiatives. The first such initiative was the treatment-IND mechanism, established in 1987, which allows expanded access to some experimental treatments before they are approved. Under the treatment-IND regulations, FDA may approve the distribution of an investigational drug outside the context of controlled clinical trials to treat patients with serious or immediately life-threatening diseases for which no comparable or satisfactory alternative therapy is available [21 CFR § 312.34(a)]. For this purpose, FDA defines a disease, including a stage in the progression of a disease, to be *immediately life-threatening* if "there is a reasonable likelihood that death will occur within a matter of months" or "if premature death is likely without early treatment" [21 CFR § 312.34(b)(3)(ii)]. Whether a disease or a particular stage of a disease is *serious* depends on "its impact on such factors as survival, day-to-day functioning, or the likelihood that the disease, if left untreated, will progress to a more serious one" (FDA, 1992a). The standard for

FDA approval of a treatment IND in the case of a "life-threatening disease," in turn, is whether the "available scientific evidence, taken as a whole," provides a "reasonable basis" for concluding that the drug "may be effective for its intended use in the intended patient population" and would not expose patients to an "unreasonable and significant additional risk of illness and injury" [21 CFR § 312.34(b)(3)(i)]. For a "serious disease," the standard is whether there is sufficient evidence of safety and effectiveness to support treatment use [21 CFR § 312.34(b)(2)].

Most of the customary IND procedural requirements apply to treatment INDs, including informed-consent requirements and prohibitions on preapproval promotion or other commercialization of experimental treatments (although companies normally may charge to cover costs) [21 CFR §§ 312.34(c), 312.7(d)(2)]. In addition, the drug sponsor is expected to continue conventional clinical trials and to pursue marketing approval of the drug with "due diligence" [21 CFR § 312.34(b)(iv)]. Among the products that FDA has approved for treatment-IND status are drugs for the treatment of hairy-cell leukemia, AIDS and AIDS related conditions, Alzheimer's disease, multiple sclerosis, respiratory distress syndrome in infants, Gaucher's disease, obsessive-compulsive disorder, Parkinson's disease, and ovarian cancer (FDA, 1993c).

Although the treatment-IND program was designed primarily for patients who could benefit from earlier access to promising experimental drugs, it theoretically offers potential benefits from a sponsor's perspective as well. It allows recovery of developmental costs earlier in the process than might otherwise be possible. It also offers the chance to familiarize patients, prescribers, and payers with a product earlier in the process, and this can facilitate the formal introduction and initial marketing of the product (as long as the sponsor keeps applicable restrictions on preapproval promotion and commercialization in mind). Given that drug addiction should qualify as a serious, and even a life-threatening, disease for treatment-IND purposes,

The committee recommends that the FDA make the treatment-IND route available for anti-addiction medications.

A second mechanism, known as parallel track, also extends the availability of investigational treatments. Although it is now limited to AIDS patients, parallel track might be adapted to a program tailored to meet the needs of drug-addicted patients in combating addiction. Under parallel track, "promising" investigational agents may be provided to AIDS patients who are not able to take standard therapy or for whom standard therapy is no longer effective and who are not able to participate in clinical trials (U.S. DHHS, 1992). Parallel-track drugs are thus distributed entirely outside the controlled clinical-trial framework, although they must be under a study protocol and data on safety and side effects must still be collected (U.S. DHHS, 1992). The evidence of effectiveness needed for a parallel-track drug is less than that generally required for a treatment IND; the parallel-track standard is "promising evidence of efficacy" combined with evidence that the drug is "reasonably safe" (U.S. DHHS, 1992). In reviewing a parallel-track proposal, FDA looks at such factors as evidence of a lack of satisfactory alternative therapy and the possible impact of the parallel-track study on the controlled trials that will be the primary source of evidence of the drug's efficacy (U.S. DHHS, 1992).[1]

With its goals of reaching patients beyond the scope of standard therapy or conventional clinical trials, parallel track provides a prototype for expanding access to treatment to addicted patients, who share some general characteristics with AIDS patients. For example, it is often difficult to find drug-addicted individuals who qualify as subjects for controlled clinical trials. Both population groups include members who might take other drugs that confound the interpretation of controlled clinical trials. For AIDS patients, the issue is exposure to other treatments; for drug-addicted patients, the issue is polydrug use. In addition, as with AIDS, there can be important ethical and recruitment issues with respect to placebo (or no-treatment) controls. Furthermore, a parallel-track procedure that would reach addicted individuals who might otherwise fall outside the system (at least at the testing stage) might further the important public-policy goals of preventing and treating drug addiction. Therefore,

The committee recommends that FDA include medications for drug addiction in the parallel-track mechanism.

Another important development aimed at speeding the drug-approval process is FDA's accelerated-approval program. Adopted in its final form in December 1992, accelerated approval is available for drugs that offer "meaningful therapeutic benefit compared to existing treatment" for "serious or life-threatening illnesses" and whose approval is to be based on evidence of the drug's effect "on a surrogate end point that reasonably suggests clinical benefit or . . . on a clinical

---

[1]In addition, some formal IND requirements do not necessarily apply, most notably supervision by an institutional review board. However, the parallel-track policy statement contemplates a national panel of "human subjects" to protect patients in parallel-track programs. At least in theory, individual patients seeking access to parallel-track treatments must satisfy a fairly detailed and stringent set of entry criteria designed to exclude patients who could take standard approved treatments.

end point other than survival or irreversible morbidity" (FDA, 1992b).[2] Such approval will be conditioned on completion of postmarketing clinical studies to "verify and describe [the drug's] clinical benefit and to resolve remaining uncertainty about the relationship of the surrogate end point to clinical benefit" (21 CFR § 314.510). Drugs approved under the accelerated procedure are also subject to a streamlined procedure for withdrawal of approval, e.g., if a postmarketing clinical study fails to verify clinical benefit (21 CFR § 314.530). Thus,

The committee recommends that, to the extent that a valid end point for the effectiveness of an anti-addiction medication might be established, accelerated approval be available.

The committee is impressed that these newer administrative mechanisms for drug distribution under INDs and for more rapid approval are properly applicable to anti-addiction medications, but it notes that FDA has not included anti-addiction medications in its public statements or written examples in the *Federal Register* related to these new policies.

We encourage the commissioner of FDA to announce clearly (in public statements and the *Federal Register*) that treatment IND, parallel track, and accelerated approval are applicable to anti-addiction medications as an incentive to private investment in this field.

Market Exclusivity and Orphan Drug Status

Other potential sources of incentives for anti-addiction drug development are the various statutory exclusivity provisions. The 1984 Drug Price Competition and Patent Term Restoration Act (DPC-PTR Act, Public Law 98-417), which amended the FDCA, gives a sponsor of a drug that is a new chemical entity 5 years of market exclusivity after NDA approval, during which time no other sponsor may submit an abbreviated application for a generic version of the same drug [FDCA §§ 505(c)(3)(D)(ii), 505(j)(4)(D)(ii)]. Manufacturers of drugs approved for a new indication are granted 3 years of exclusivity for the new indication if new clinical tests were "necessary" to support the approval [FDCA §§ 505(c)(3)(D)(iv), 505(j)(4)(D)(iv)]. In addition, the DPC-PTR Act allows a

---

[2]Surrogate end points are clinical or laboratory measurements that correlate with patient benefit, such as $CD4^+$ blood-cell counts as a basis for assessing the efficacy of AIDS drugs or reduction in blood pressure as a predictor of decreased mortality or morbidity due to hypertensive cardiovascular disease (e.g., stroke, heart failure, and myocardial infarction).

manufacturer to obtain an extension to its patent term for a portion of the term lost while the product was in regulatory review if the sponsor pursued its marketing application with due diligence (35 USC § 156).

A separate basis for exclusivity is the Orphan Drug Act (Public Law 97-414, FDCA §§ 525-528). This law, enacted in 1983 and amended several times, is intended to encourage the development of drugs needed to treat rare diseases whose potential sales might not justify funding of the animal and clinical trials needed to bring products to approval. The standard for orphan status is whether a drug is intended to treat a "rare disease or condition," i.e., a disease or condition that affects fewer than 200,000 persons in the United States or that affects more than 200,000 but for which there is no reasonable expectation of recovering development costs from sales in the United States.

To obtain orphan exclusivity, a sponsor must first request and obtain FDA designation of its drug as an orphan drug. The request, which must be filed before the sponsor submits its marketing application for the product and be granted before the marketing application is approved, must include a description of the rare disease or condition for which the drug is being investigated, the reasons why the drug is needed for the disease or condition, a description of the drug and a discussion of its scientific rationale, and documentation of the rarity of the disease or condition within the meaning of the statute (21 CFR § 316.20). A drug that has been designated an orphan is entitled to marketing exclusivity for 7 years after approval, during which time FDA may not approve another sponsor's application for the same drug for the approved orphan indication, apart from specified exceptions.[3]

In addition to market exclusivity, an orphan-drug manufacturer may apply for special FDA orphan research grants and contracts and is eligible for tax credits for the costs of clinical trials conducted in the United States. Also, FDA, if asked, must provide the sponsor with written protocol recommendations, and the statute instructs FDA to encourage open-label studies so that patients needing the drug have access to it (FDCA §§ 525, 528; 26 USC § 44H).

Several sponsors of anti-addiction drugs already have taken advantage of the orphan-drug provisions. For example, LAAM was granted orphan status for the treatment of heroin addicted patients suitable for maintenance on opiate agonists, as was Du Pont's Trexan® (naltrexone) for maintenance of the opiate-free state in detoxified formerly opiate-addicted persons by blocking the effects of exogenously administered opiates (FDA, 1994). In addition, Pharmavene Inc. obtained an orphan-drug designation for its product butrylcholinesterase, which

---

[3]These exceptions include inability of an orphan-exclusivity holder to ensure a supply of the drug [FDCA § 528(b)(1)] and demonstration by a second sponsor that its version of the product is clinically superior to the orphan-exclusivity holder's version [21 CFR § 316.3(b)(13)(ii)].

is in testing for increasing the clearance of toxic blood concentrations of cocaine produced by a drug overdose (FDA, 1993a). Although the sponsors of LAAM took advantage of the provisions of the Orphan Drug Act, the fact that other manufacturers of anti-addiction drugs now in development have not obtained orphan status might indicate that additional incentives are needed. Legislation that would have granted orphan-drug incentives specifically to manufacturers of anti-addiction drugs was proposed in 1989 and 1990 but was not enacted [S. 1711, 101st Cong., 1st Sess. (1989); S. 2649, 101st Cong., 2d Sess. (1990); S 2650, 101st Cong., 2d Sess. (1990)]. This issue is further explored in Chapter 9 and a recommendation is made.

FDA Guidelines on Evaluation of
Anti-Addiction Drugs

The FDA has written draft guidelines intended to assist manufacturers in developing new anti-addiction drugs (FDA, 1992c). The draft document entitled "Guidelines for the Development and Evaluation of Drugs for the Treatment of Psychoactive Substance Use Disorders" is circulating within FDA and is not yet publicly available.[4] The guidelines address such issues as appropriate clinical end points, clinical-trial methods, the use of adolescents in clinical trials (an important issue, given the age of the drug-addiction patient population), polydrug abuse, and the greater potential for abuse of prescription drugs by drug users than by the rest of the population (FDA, 1992c).

Several of those issues require special mention. The question of appropriate clinical end points in establishing the effectiveness of anti-addiction drugs has long been debated for a number of reasons, including the nature of the patient population, the use of women and pregnant drug users in clinical trials, the ethics of using placebo or no-treatment controls, and the difficulties of measuring abstinence and recidivism. In principle, the ideal clinical end point would be cessation of drug addiction without the need for maintenance therapy with a treatment drug. However, reduction in, rather than outright cessation of, use of the illegal drug in question might also be a suitable end point. Cessation or reduction, in turn, can be measured through biological tests, self-reporting of use, measurement of money spent on drugs, or a challenge test. Other possible end points might be: retention time in therapy, severity of dependence, withdrawal symptoms or drug-abuse toxicities, patient craving for the drug, illegal activities involvement related to drug use, employment or family status, and mortality or morbidity.

---

[4]The committee received a copy of the guidelines for developing and evaluating anti-addiction medications after the publication of the preliminary report (March 1994).

Another guideline issue concerns the evidence required for evaluation of the safety and effectiveness of anti-addiction drugs. For example, although LAAM had been the subject of over 20 studies from 1969 through the early 1980s, FDA required the completion of a "usage" study before approval (FDA, 1993b). It was concerned about the application of LAAM to the current drug-addict population and whether the directions for use would ensure successful treatment, i.e., in methadone (now narcotic) treatment clinics (FDA, 1992d). The study was an uncontrolled "open-label" (unblinded) trial designed so that drug-addicted individuals were permitted to come in directly and participate. Efficacy was measured by retention rate and "dirty urine" and safety by serious adverse reactions (FDA, 1992d). To resolve the ethical questions raised by a placebo control, the study used historical controls that were based on comparable data on methadone use (FDA, 1992d). Thus although FDA is likely to require some clinical information on "real-world" conditions of use for particular anti-addiction drugs, it appears to be flexible in accepting nontraditional trial designs to obtain such information.

The committee is impressed that the guidelines on efficacy end points and approval requirements are valuable to drug sponsors in planning their drug-development programs. Clinical guidelines diminish the uncertainty faced by private sponsors and can serve as an incentive to develop anti-addiction medications. Therefore,

The committee recommends that FDA make publicly available the draft guidelines for developing and evaluating anti-addiction medications, seek open comment from the private sector and academic experts, and then complete and publish those guidelines in a timely way.

DRUG ENFORCEMENT ADMINISTRATION

Scheduling

FDA's approval of an anti-addiction drug does not necessarily end the regulatory requirements for marketing the drug. If the drug is a narcotic itself or is subject to abuse, as are methadone and LAAM, it is subject to regulation as a controlled substance by DEA. For those drugs, there is another step before marketing can occur. When FDA reviews a new drug product with a potential for abuse, it must notify DEA (Controlled Substances Act § 201(f); 21 USC § 801(f); 21 CFR 314.104). FDA requires that an NDA include a section assessing the drug product's abuse liability (FDA, 1990). During the review process, FDA, with the assistance of the Drug Abuse Advisory Committee and input from

NIDA (FDA, 1985), makes a scheduling recommendation to DEA using the criteria outlined in the Controlled Substances Act [CSA §§201(b), (c); 21 USC §§ 811(b), (c)].[5] Under the CSA, a drug with a potential for abuse is placed into one of five schedules, depending on the magnitude of the potential for abuse, whether the drug has accepted medical uses, and the extent to which abuse of the drug will lead to physical or psychological dependence.[6] The restrictions and requirements that apply depend on the schedule into which a particular drug product falls. Congress made the initial scheduling determinations in the statute; DEA has authority to make scheduling decisions for new drugs not covered in the statute and to reschedule drugs under some circumstances (CSA §§ 201, 202; 21 USC §§ 811, 812).

After receipt of FDA's recommendation, DEA makes its initial scheduling determination and publishes it as a proposed rule in the *Federal Register*, waits for comments, and then issues its final rule. This might occur before or after FDA approval. In the mid-1980s, FDA routinely issued NDA "approvable" letters for drugs proposed for scheduling. In 1986, FDA changed its policy regarding NDA approvals for drugs pending scheduling and issued final "approval" letters with the addition of a statement that the drug could not be marketed until it was scheduled by DEA. The result was that the "clock" measuring time before patent expiration, for DPC-PTR Act purposes, was started, even though the drug was not able to be marketed. Under current FDA policy, issuance of a

---

[5]The criteria include the scientific evidence of the drug's pharmacologic effect, if known; the state of scientific knowledge regarding the drug; the risk, if any, to the public health; the drug's psychic or physiologic dependence liability; whether it is an immediate precursor of a substance already controlled; the scientific and medical considerations involved in the drug's actual or relative potential for abuse; its history and current pattern of abuse; and the scope, duration, and significance of abuse.

[6]Specifically, a Schedule I drug has a high potential for abuse, has no accepted medical use in treatment in the United States, and there is a lack of accepted safety for use of the drug under medical supervision; a Schedule II drug has a high potential for abuse and has an accepted medical use in treatment in the United States or an accepted medical use with severe restrictions, and its abuse might lead to severe psychologic or physical dependence; a Schedule III drug has a lower potential for abuse than a Schedule I or II drug and has an accepted medical use in treatment in the United States, and its abuse might lead to moderate or low physical dependence or high psychologic dependence; a Schedule IV drug has a lower potential for abuse than a Schedule III drug and has an accepted medical use in treatment in the United States, and its abuse might lead to less physical or psychologic dependence than a Schedule III drug; and a Schedule V drug has a lower potential for abuse than a Schedule IV drug and has an accepted medical use in treatment in the United States, and its abuse might lead to less physical or psychologic abuse than a Schedule IV drug [CSA § 202(b)].

final approval letter seems to permit sale under the Food, Drug and Cosmetic Act without restriction, and no provision of the CSA applies to a drug that is not controlled under that Act.

Drug manufacturers have complained about the delay in DEA scheduling. Typically, scheduling can take from several weeks up to 2 months after approval of an NDA by FDA. For example, in the case of LAAM, DEA published its proposed decision to transfer the product from Schedule I to Schedule II in April 1993, before the NDA was approved. A 30-day comment period was set, and the final rule was issued on August 18, 1993, about 5 weeks after the NDA was approved (DEA, 1993).

The lag at DEA, if it becomes substantial, has practical implications for anti-addiction drugs, with respect to lost marketing time. As stated above, pioneer drug manufacturers might be eligible for patent-term extension to allow them to recoup the time lost during regulatory review. In calculating the review period for controlled substances, however, FDA does not count the time lost after approval of an NDA through scheduling by DEA (FDA, 1988); this time is unrecoverable by the manufacturer.

The committee recommends that DEA review time be counted as part of the regulatory process for purposes of patent-term extension for controlled substances.

To accomplish this, any of the following three options could be implemented:

- **Amend the DPC-PTR Act.**
- **Concurrent DEA scheduling and FDA approval, in the final stages of drug review.**
- **Unilateral FDA reversion to its earlier policy of issuing NDA "approvable" letters for drugs proposed for scheduling.**

The committee has reviewed the issue of scheduling at the state level in Chapter 8 and offers an additional recommendation regarding this issue.

Quotas

If a drug is scheduled by DEA as a controlled substance, its manufacture is heavily regulated by DEA. Specifically, DEA must set aggregate and individual annual production quotas for Schedule I and II drugs (CSA § 306; 21 USC § 826), a process in which FDA also plays a role (21 CFR Part 1303). In particular, FDA must report to DEA the "results of studies and investigations of quantities of narcotic drugs or other drugs subject to control under [the CSA], together with reserves of such drugs, that are necessary to supply the normal and emergency medical and scientific requirements of the United States . . . not later than the first of April of each year" [Public Health Service Act § 302(a); 42 USC § 242(a)]. With FDA's recommendation in mind, DEA establishes yearly aggregate production quotas for each Schedule I and II drug to meet "the estimated medical, scientific, research, and industrial needs of the United States, for lawful export requirements, and for the establishment and maintenance of reserve stocks" [CSA § 306(a); 21 USC 21 826(a)].

Although the purpose of the DEA quota system is to prevent inappropriate diversion of controlled substances, it also has the effect of restricting a manufacturer's ability to manufacture and sell its product. Quotas may also affect manufacturing costs, because optimal batch sizes may exceed quota limits. Furthermore, the scheduling of a drug imposes substantial restrictions on the prescribing of the drug by physicians. Those factors combine to make the scheduling of a drug an important disincentive to developing a drug with addiction potential.

Regulatory Authority Over Anti-Addiction Drugs In Development

DEA's jurisdiction over a drug undergoing clinical investigation for an anti-addiction indication depends on whether the drug is a controlled substance. If the drug is a new chemical entity that has not been scheduled under the CSA, it is not necessarily under DEA jurisdiction at the clinical-trial stage, even though it might later be scheduled. FDA is not required to notify DEA about a new drug that is not yet (but that ultimately might be) scheduled until it receives an NDA for the drug, which will presumably be after clinical trials have been completed [CSA § 201(f); 21 USC § 811(f)]. However, FDA could apprise DEA of the drug at an earlier stage in the process if it thought that the drug had a potential for abuse, in which case it is possible that the drug could be scheduled while still in clinical trials or even earlier. If the investigational drug is already a controlled substance (as was LAAM), then it will by definition be subject to DEA jurisdiction while in clinical trials. Although holders of INDs for controlled substances are exempt from some DEA requirements that parallel FDA requirements, DEA still maintains substantial authority over the manufacture, distribution, and research use of controlled substances, subjecting researchers of new anti-addiction drugs to a dual regulatory scheme.

The CSA and DEA's regulations require that persons conducting clinical research with any controlled substance register with DEA [CSA §302(a)(1); 21 USC §822 (a)(1); see also 21 CFR §§ 1301.21, 1301.22(a), 1301.22(b)(5)], keep specific kinds of records [CSA § 307(a),(b); 21 USC § 827(a), (b)], and periodically report to DEA [CSA § 307(d); 21 USC § 827(d)]. Holders of INDs for controlled substances must register with DEA but are exempt from the CSA's recordkeeping requirements (CSA § 307(c)(2)(A); 21 USC § 827(c)(2)(A); see 21 CFR Part 1304). In particular, 21 CFR § 1304.03(e) provides that a DEA registrant operating under an IND who "maintains records in accordance with [the FDCA] is not required to keep records if he notifies [DEA] of the name, address, and registration number of the establishment maintaining such records." FDA requires, however, that a sponsor or investigator make its FDA-mandated records pertaining to shipment, delivery, receipt, and disposition of the drug available to DEA for inspection and copying at DEA's request [21 CFR § 312.58(b)]. In addition, FDA regulations mandate that investigators and sponsors in clinical trials using controlled substances take special precautions, including storage of the drug in a secure place with limited access, to prevent theft or inappropriate diversion [21 CFR §§ 312.69, 312.58(b)]. This regulation is consistent with Section 307(f) of the CSA, 21 USC § 827(f), which requires FDA to promulgate rules to "insure the security and accountability of controlled substances" used in clinical investigations.

There is, however, no corresponding exemption from the reporting requirements under the CSA [CSA § 307(d); 21 USC § 827(d)]. In addition, because a DEA registration for research with controlled substances also authorizes the manufacture and distribution of such substances (within defined limits) [21 CFR § 1301.22(b)(3) for Schedule I and (b)(5) for Schedules II-V] if a researcher engages in either activity, he or she must comply with the recordkeeping and reporting requirements for manufacturers and distributors [21 CFR § 1304.03(a)]. Thus, for example, the holder of an IND for a controlled substance that also manufactures it must report data on the acquisition and reduction of the substance from inventory monthly (unless it receives permission from DEA to report more or less often) and data on the status of year-end inventory annually if the controlled substance is in Schedule I or II, is a narcotic in Schedules III, IV, or V, or is a listed psychotropic substance in Schedule III or IV (21 CFR § 1304.35).

In addition, DEA requires that protocols for research with Schedule I controlled substances be submitted to it for approval and requires researchers using Schedule I substances to identify in their registration applications the extent to which the research will also involve manufacture or importation (21 CFR §§ 1301.32(a)(6), 1301.33). This does not, however, apply to clinical investigations under an IND. In those cases, the sponsor need only submit to DEA a copy of its IND with a statement of the security provisions for storing and dispensing the drug to prevent inappropriate diversion [21 CFR § 1301.33(b)]. In either case, FDA has the ultimate authority to approve the study, either under the provisions of the FDCA pertaining to INDs or, for research protocols not under an IND, under 21 CFR § 1301.42, which requires DEA to forward applications for registration for research with Schedule I substances to FDA. In making its determination as to the merits of the study under the latter provision, FDA must consult with DEA as to the adequacy of procedures to be taken to prevent inappropriate diversion (21 CFR § 1301.42). When an investigator wants to increase the amount of a Schedule I controlled substance that it has received approval to use, the sponsor first must submit a request to DEA; DEA then forwards the request to FDA, which may grant or deny the request, taking into account DEA's comments [21 CFR § 1301.33(c)].

The practical consequence of this dual authority over clinical research, particularly in the light of the additional complication of multiple state laws patterned after the CSA (Chapter 8), is a clinical research environment for scheduled drugs that is extraordinarily bureaucratic from the procedural point of view and unnecessarily difficult. That is especially true given the relatively small amounts of any controlled substance used in research; thus the consequences of diversion to public health would be small even if the diversion from research was substantial. The administrative effort required to cope with this complex system is discussed in Chapter 3. The difficulty of conducting clinical research is also cited in the private sector as an important deterrent to R&D investment (Chapter 9). Even if the new drug under study is not scheduled, the comparative agent in positively controlled studies of the drug (which might well be the pivotal studies for FDA approval) could be a controlled substance like methadone; this would trigger the complex dual system of regulation. Finally, studies to optimize the dose or dose schedule of a new drug and to extend the use to new patient populations, such as pregnant women and adolescents, are typically done after marketing, which means after the drug is scheduled. All studies of this type are vastly more difficult on scheduled drugs and therefore, as a practical matter, tend not to be done.

> **The committee recommends that action be taken to remove the adverse effects of DEA requirements, under the Controlled Substances Act (CSA), on clinical research investigations involving controlled substances, by holders of active FDA INDs, either by amending the CSA to exempt such investigations from applicable DEA regulations or by the alternative administrative and regulatory measures:**
>
> > • **The development of a Memorandum of Understanding between FDA and DEA governing the matter of dual authority over clinical research to provide exemption from DEA reporting requirements.**
> > • **DEA revision of 21 CFR 1301.33 and parallel regulations to provide that protocols, drug security, recordkeeping, production controls, reporting, and other requirements would be governed by**

the FDA regulations and monitored by FDA. This would require parallel changes in FDA's IND regulations.

FDA's current provisions for control and recording the disposition of controlled substances under an IND should be adequate to address concerns of drug security and diversion.

CONCLUSIONS

The committee concludes that the complexities faced in the normal process of drug discovery and development are made even more daunting and costly by the multitude of regulations and clinical research constraints imposed by FDA and DEA in the development of anti-addiction medications. Thus, the committee has offered recommendations with the intent of easing the regulatory disincentives to the pharmaceutical industry and expediting the availability of new pharmacotherapies for heroin and cocaine addicts.

REFERENCES

Agersborg HPK. 1993. Characteristics of Development Candidates and Overview of Development Process. Presentation at the Pharmaceutical Manufacturers Association Basic Course on Drug Development. May 23–26, 1993, San Francisco.

DEA (Drug Enforcement Administration). 1993. Schedules of controlled substances: transfer of levo-alpha-acetyl-methadol from Schedule I to Schedule II. August 18, 1993. Federal Register 58(158):43795.

DiMasi JA, Hansen RW, Grabowski HG, Lasagna L. 1991. Cost of innovation in the pharmaceutical industry. Journal of Health Economics 10:107-142.

FDA (Food and Drug Administration). 1985. Memorandum of Understanding with National Institute on Drug Abuse. May 1, 1985.

FDA (Food and Drug Administration). 1988. Patent Term Restoration regulations. March 7, 1988. Federal Register 53(44):7298–7309.

FDA (Food and Drug Administration). 1990. Draft Guidelines for Abuse Liability Assessment. July 20, 1990. Drug Abuse Advisory Committee.

FDA (Food and Drug Administration). 1992a. New Drug, Antibiotic, and Biological Drug Product Regulations; Accelerated Approval. Proposed Rule. April 15, 1992. Federal Register 57:13234.

FDA (Food and Drug Administration). 1992b. New Drug, Antibiotic, and Biological Drug Product Regulations; Accelerated Approval. Final Rule. December 11, 1992. 57 Federal Register 57:58942.

FDA (Food and Drug Administration). 1992c. Drug Abuse Advisory Committee Transcript of Meeting No. 24, 9–30. December 10, 1992.

FDA (Food and Drug Administration). 1992d. Summary Basis for Approval for LAAM, NDA #20-315, Medical Officer Review of LAAM Usage Study.

FDA (Food and Drug Administration). 1993a. Approved Drug Products with Therapeutic Equivalent Evaluations, 13th ed. Section 3.6, Orphan Drug Product Designations. Washington, DC: U.S. Government Printing Office.

FDA (Food and Drug Administration). 1993b. Levo-alpha-acetyl-methanol (LAAM) in maintenance: revision of conditions for use in the treatment of narcotic addiction. July 20, 1993. Federal Register 58: 38704–38711.

FDA (Food and Drug Administration). 1993c. Treatment Investigational New Drugs Allowed to Proceed (June 22, 1987–Nov. 5, 1993).

FDA (Food and Drug Administration). 1994. Cumulative List of Orphan Product Designations and Approval. December 31, 1994. FDA Office of Orphan Products Development.

Grabowski HG, Vernon JM. 1990. Unpublished appendix to: A New Look at the Returns and Risks to Pharmaceutical R&D. Durham, NC: Duke University Department of Economics. As cited in: Office of Technology Assessment (OTA). 1993. Pharmaceutical R & D: Costs, Risks and Rewards. Washington, DC: Government Printing Office. OTA-H-522.

Kaitin KI, Bryant NR, Lasagna L. 1993. The role of the research-based pharmaceutical industry in medical progress in the United States. Journal of Clinical Pharmacology 33:412–417.

Knoop SJ, Worden DE. 1988. The pharmaceutical drug development process: an overview. Drug Information Journal 22:259–268.

NIDA (National Institute on Drug Abuse). 1990. NIDA's Medications Development Program. NIDA Notes Summer:31.

OTA (Office of Technology Assessment). 1993. Pharmaceutical R & D: Costs, Risks and Rewards. Washington, DC: Government Printing Office. OTA-H-522.

PMA (Pharmaceutical Manufacturers Association). 1993a. Drug Discovery. Industry Issue Brief 26. Washington, DC: PMA.

PMA (Pharmaceutical Manufacturers Association). 1993b. Federal-Industry Drug Research Collaboration. Industry Issue Brief 8. Washington, DC: PMA.

Rapaka RS, Hawks RL, eds. 1993. Medications Development: Drug Discovery, Databases, and Computer-Aided Drug Design. Rockville, MD: NIDA. NIDA Research Monograph 134.

Spilker B. 1989. Multinational Drug Companies: Issues in Drug Discovery and Development. New York: Raven Press.

Spilker B, Cuatrecasas P. 1990. Inside the Drug Industry. Barcelona: Prous Science.

U.S. DHHS (U.S. Department of Health and Human Services, Public Health Service). 1992. Expanded Availability of Investigation New Drugs Through a Parallel Track Mechanism for People with AIDS and Other HIV-Related Disease. Parallel Track Policy Statement. April 15, 1992. Federal Register 57:13250.

Wesson DR, Ling W. 1991. Medications in the treatment of addictive disease. Journal of Psychoactive Drugs 23:365–369.

Wiggins SN. 1987. The Cost of Developing a New Drug. Washington, DC: Pharmaceutical Manufacturers Association.

8

State Laws and Regulations

State laws and regulations affect the discovery, development, and marketing of anti-addiction medications, especially if the medication is a controlled substance. Current medications to treat opiate addiction (methadone and levo-alpha-acetylmethadol or LAAM) are Schedule II narcotics that are tightly regulated, not only under the federal Controlled Substances Act (CSA; P.L. 91-513) and the Narcotic Addict Treatment Act (NATA; P.L. 93-281) but also under companion state laws. All states and the District of Columbia have regulations that are counterparts to the comprehensive federal regulatory structure for controlled substances (Chapter 7). Rather than set the upper boundaries of state regulation, federal laws and regulations establish minimum requirements above which states may impose stricter or additional requirements. As a result, there are significant variations in statutes from state to state, and numerous differences between federal and state provisions (NCJA, 1991). If the medications being developed are controlled substances, state laws can have as great a practical effect as the federal laws.

This chapter examines the effect of state laws and regulations on the use of controlled substances in research and treatment, and it discusses the effects of state laws and regulations on private-sector development of new anti-addiction medications that are controlled substances.

173

STATE REGULATORY LANDSCAPE

State and federal controlled substances acts (CSAs) are designed primarily to govern the possession, use, sale, distribution, and manufacture of medications that have a potential for abuse. Most state CSAs contain regulatory mechanisms, terminology, and provisions similar to those contained in the federal CSA.

During the discovery and development of any drug, pharmaceutical companies must interact continuously with the relevant federal agencies. Additional federal interactions are required when developing a Schedule I or II narcotic (Chapter 7), and pharmaceutical companies developing such products also are faced with the regulatory authority of each state. Some states have established comprehensive laws and regulations for controlled substances that address scheduling and rescheduling of medications; the conduct of clinical research (including researcher registration, clinic licensure, clinical trial protocol approvals); registrations and licenses for manufacturers, distributors, prescribers, and dispensers; the administration of treatment centers (including approval and registration, record keeping, administrative policies and procedures, product storage, and licensing of practitioners); and restriction on dispensing, labeling, and advertising. A failure to understand the regulatory framework in each state can lead to significant delays in clinical research development, marketing and use of a new anti-addiction medication, as shown by the LAAM case study presented later in this chapter. Any perceived delay in a return on investment to a pharmaceutical company can influence the decision to develop a new anti-addiction medication. Inasmuch as this area is already perceived as a marginal business investment, the additional overlay of the state laws and regulations and the resulting delays can negatively influence manufacturers' decisions to enter the field.

The following sections present an overview of a range of selected state regulations that affect anti-addiction medications development. State scheduling, treatment, and clinical research regulations are described.

Scheduling

The federal CSA places all substances into one of five schedules (Chapter 7). Placement is based on the substance's medical efficacy, safety, potential for abuse and diversion, and physical and psychological dependence liability; substances placed in one schedule can be rescheduled (21 USC § 811) as new information becomes available.

Although some states have adopted schedules identical to the federal schedules (basing their action on the uniform model developed by the National Conference of Commissioners on Uniform State Laws), some reschedule controlled substances independently of the federal government and more restrictively. The process of state scheduling of new drugs and revising the schedules of existing drugs occurs in three ways: automatic rescheduling, administrative rule-making, or, in many states, by new legislation. In any case, the process does not usually begin until a drug has been scheduled or rescheduled at the federal level (Chapter 7).

In many states (including Texas, Illinois, and New Jersey), the scheduling procedure is triggered automatically by a federal scheduling determination, and the medication is presumptively placed into the same schedule as the federal schedule. The entire process can be accomplished in about 30 days. In those states, however, public hearings can be held in case of objections, often slowing the process. In other states (including Pennsylvania, New York, California), there is no formal linkage between the state scheduling process and the federal process, nor is there any time limit on the state scheduling process. In those states, independent action by a state body (either a state regulatory agency or the state legislature) is necessary to begin the scheduling process.

States differ as to whether the legislature or a regulatory agency (or both) is primarily responsible for scheduling. For example, in South Carolina, Rhode Island, and Tennessee the scheduling determination is made by a regulatory agency (usually with an explicit provision for a legislative override); in New York and California, state legislative action is required. In other states (Iowa, Hawaii, Mississippi), the legislature and the state regulatory agencies are involved in the scheduling and rescheduling process.

Variations in the scheduling process can have a substantial effect on the marketing of a new medication. The fact that each state has its own scheduling mechanism creates a daunting set of tasks for prospective manufacturers. The potential for serious delay is real, particularly in states that require legislative action, because not all state legislatures meet in continuous session (for example, in 1994 only 38 state legislatures met in regular session). Such delays add a significant obstacle to pharmaceutical companies in calculating a return on the initial investment. In particular, the LAAM scheduling experience could dissuade companies as they consider developing portfolios of future anti-addiction medications (see LAAM case study below).

While state inactivity is rescheduling can result in long delays in moving a drug from schedule I (under state Controlled Substances Acts) to schedules II to V, this situation is brought about in part by the current federal policy of interpreting "currently accepted medical use in treatment in the United States" (for purposes of scheduling under the Controlled Substances Act) as requiring NDA (new drug application) approval. A consequence of this policy is that the regulatory process at the federal level is prolonged for all newly approved drugs that are controlled substances (Chapter 7); this regulatory delay can become years when the rescheduling process requires both state and federal action and cannot begin until NDA approval, e.g., LAAM. The committee believes that the public health would be best served by an interpretation of the "currently accepted medical use" clause in the Controlled Substances Act that would recognize the use in humans under an IND (investigational new drug) and permit the scheduling process to begin at the time of NDA submission. The information required for scheduling a drug is already required to be in a self-contained section of the NDA. That section could be reviewed on a fast-track basis by the Food and Drug Administration (FDA), and a scheduling recommendation could be sent to the Drug Enforcement Administration (DEA) well ahead of NDA approval. Scheduling could be done contingent upon final FDA approval. That approach would permit states to reschedule schedule I drugs closer in time to final FDA approval, minimizing delays such as the one now affecting LAAM, and have no negative drug control implications. Furthermore, it would remove a significant regulatory disincentive at the federal level that affects all scheduled drugs, not just schedule I substances.

The committee recommends that the Office of National Drug Control Policy (ONDCP) direct DEA, in consultation with FDA and the National Institute on Drug Abuse (NIDA), to revise its policy on determining when a drug has a currently accepted medical use in treatment so that, for new therapeutic drugs that are also controlled substances, the process of scheduling can begin as soon as possible after submission of the NDA.

Treatment

Each state is responsible for approving narcotic treatment programs and for monitoring those programs for compliance with state regulations. State treatment regulations must be at least as restrictive as federal regulations, but more stringent regulations are allowed. State approval of narcotic treatment programs is a prerequisite for federal approval, and individual states can recommend to the FDA that a program's approval be revoked for noncompliance [21 CFR § 291.505(h)(2)] (SAMHSA, 1992).[1] Any new anti-addiction medication that is

---

[1]In that case, FDA's Center for Drug Evaluation and Research (CDER) will notify the treatment program, which will be given the opportunity to respond in an informal hearing or in writing within 10 days [21 CFR § 291.505(h)(2)]. If the explanation offered is unacceptable, the FDA commissioner must provide the opportunity for a hearing, render a decision, and notify all appropriate authorities, including the state [21 CFR § 291.505(h)(3)]. FDA, however, has no authority to grant an appeal if the revocation is based on state law or regulation [21 CFR § 291.505(h)(5)].

a narcotic will be required, under federal regulations, to be distributed through approved narcotic treatment programs. The states must not only schedule or reschedule the new medication, but they must also amend their treatment regulations to accommodate the new product before granting approval for its use in treatment.

Until recently, methadone was the only medication approved for use in narcotic treatment programs, and state regulations were written only for methadone maintenance treatment. Once a new anti-addiction medication receives FDA approval for the treatment of drug dependence, the states must amend their methadone regulations before it is used in a program. Thus, under the current regulatory landscape, there could be substantial delays before any newly approved anti-addiction medication actually reaches the patient population. In fact, not even methadone maintenance therapy is available in all states (SAMHSA, 1992).

A sample of state treatment regulations, discussed below, illustrates the complexities faced by pharmaceutical companies as they determine the feasibility of developing a new medication and the probability of success that a new anti-addiction medication will deliver an adequate return on investment.

Admission Criteria

In California, individuals may not be admitted to a narcotic maintenance treatment program unless they are currently addicted, have a 2-year addiction history, and possess evidence of two earlier failures in withdrawal treatments other than with methadone [California Code of Regulations, Title 9 § 10270(b)]. California also imposes a 2-year limit on treatment unless a physician certifies that additional treatment is medically necessary [California Code of Regulations, Title 9 § 10410(a)]. In practice, almost all programs routinely receive permission to exceed this limitation. By contrast, federal regulations require only a 1-year history of addiction, which is the norm in other states, such as New York [21 CFR § 291.505(d)(1)(i)]. New York also requires documented proof that a prospective patient has attempted detoxification or drug-free treatment at least twice [New York Compilation of Codes, Rules, and Regulations, Title 14 § 1040.5(d)].

Staffing Requirements

State staffing requirements for narcotic treatment programs span a wide range of approaches. New York specifies that each program employ one full-time physician for every 300 patients. Two full-time nurses are required for the first

300 patients, and thereafter another full-time nurse is needed for each additional 100 patients or fraction thereof. One full-time case worker is required to counsel every 50 patients (New York Compilation of Codes, Rules, and Regulations, Title 14 § 1040.15). California requires one physician for every 200 patients in a maintenance program, and one counselor for every 40 patients [California Code of Regulations, Title 9 § 10100(b)]. Massachusetts requires one full-time physician or nurse for the first 300 patients, and one nurse or physician's assistant for each additional 300 patients (Massachusetts Bureau of Substance Abuse Services, no date given). All clinics are required by federal regulations to have a licensed physician serve as the designated medical director (21 CFR § 291.505).

Patient Registries

To prevent illegal diversion of controlled medications, the federal government prohibits treatment programs from administering medications, except in an emergency situation, to "a patient who is known to be currently receiving drugs from another treatment program," and requires that patients always report to the same treatment facility, unless permission is granted otherwise [21 CFR § 291.505(e)]. New York requires the maintenance of a central registry system. Before a patient is enrolled in a treatment program, the patient's name must be submitted to a central registry, which also has information regarding patient discharges and transfers from other treatment programs (New York Compilation of Codes, Rules, and Regulations, Title 14 § 1040.4). Florida has a provision [Florida Administrative Code Rule 10E-16.003(5)] similar to New York's central registry. California attempts to prevent multiple enrollments in treatment programs through the use of a statewide database of methadone treatment participants against which prospective patients are checked (California Code of Regulations, Title 9 § 10220). If a prospective patient's initial drug screen tests positive for methadone, it is the responsibility of the treatment program's administrator to contact all other programs within a 50-mile radius (California Code of Regulations, Title 9 § 10215).

Drug Screening

Federal regulations, after initial screening, require eight random urine tests during the first year of maintenance therapy and one random test per quarter during each subsequent year. Patients who take home medications, however, must be screened monthly [21 CFR § 291.505(d)(2)(i)]. By comparison, New York requires urine testing each week during the first 3 months of treatment. If the testing shows no evidence of drug abuse, the patient need be tested only once a month [New York Compilation of Codes, Rules, and Regulations, Title 14 § 1040.12]. Monthly drug screening is the rule in California [California Code of Regulations, Title 9 § 10310(e)]; Massachusetts requires an average of 26 urine screens annually (about once every other week) (Massachusetts Bureau of Substance Abuse Services, no date given).

Medication Take-Home Policies

Federal law allows a maximum of a 2-day take-home supply of methadone after 3 months of treatment; LAAM has not yet been approved for take-home use (Chapter 5). A 3-day supply can be given to a patient who has participated in a treatment program, adhering to all its rules, for 2 years; after 3 years, a 6-day take-home supply is allowed [21 CFR § 291.505(d)(6)(v)]. Many states, however, take a stricter approach. For example, California regulations allow a 1-day take-home supply of medications after the first 3 months, but the maximum is a 3-day supply after 2 years [California Code of Regulations, Title 9 § 10375(b)]. Florida and Illinois also add further restrictions to the federal take-home policy (Florida Administrative Code Rule 10E-16.014(3)(d); Illinois Administrative Code § 2058.359). In Illinois a patient may not receive more than a 3-day take-home supply without a written exemption from the Department of Alcoholism and Substance Abuse (Illinois Administrative Code § 2058.359).

Clinical Research

Clinical research with potential new medications follows a prescribed course outlined by the FDA's IND process, and clinical trials with medications that are not controlled substances may be conducted in any state with little or no added state regulation. However, additional regulatory steps often are required for clinical trials of controlled substances, which can add further costs and delay the development process. California, for example, requires that an investigator planning to conduct research on human subjects involving a Schedule I or II substance submit the protocol to the state's research advisory panel for approval (California Health & Safety Code § 11481; Research Advisory Panel, 1993). Approval is granted for 6 months, although the investigator may request permission to extend the study. Approved research programs are subject to inspection by panel members, staff, or hired consultants, and annual progress and final reports must be submitted to the panel (Research Advisory Panel, 1993)

New York similarly requires state approval of clinical research involving Schedule I substances, and state licenses are required for anyone engaging in research with a controlled substance generally (New York Public Health Law §§ 3324 to 3329; New York Compilation of Codes, Rules, and Regulations, Title 10 § 80.36). The state also imposes record-keeping requirements for researchers who study controlled substances (New York Public Health Law § 3329; New York Compilation of Codes, Rules, and Regulations, Title 10 § 80.37).

LAAM: A CASE STUDY

The development of LAAM (marketed in the United States under the trade name ORLAAM), illustrates all too clearly how state regulations can impede the availability of an approved anti-addiction medication. LAAM is a synthetic opiate that suppresses withdrawal symptoms for up to 72 hours with minimal side effects. The main advantage of LAAM is that it is potentially more effective than methadone therapeutically. LAAM has additional advantages, when compared to methadone, such as: it must be taken less frequently (three times per week, as opposed to daily for methadone); it has a longer duration to onset of peak effect; and it produces a less euphoric effect overall. Those characteristics should provide several benefits, including alleviating overcrowding in treatment programs, reducing costs, lowering attractiveness to the illicit drug trade, and offering less potential for diversion.

LAAM was approved by FDA in July 1993 for the management of opiate dependence under an NDA sponsored by BioDevelopment Corporation (BDC). BDC has a staff of 29 people, limited financial resources, and LAAM is its only approved product. The final approval of LAAM as an anti-addiction medication was expedited through a major initiative that entailed considerable cooperation and planning among NIDA, DEA, and FDA (Chapter 3). After FDA approval, DEA rescheduled LAAM on August 18, 1993, from a Schedule I to a Schedule II narcotic under the federal CSA. Under current regulations, LAAM can be distributed only to clinics and hospitals that operate licensed narcotic treatment programs.

Since the federal rescheduling of LAAM, BDC has been working with NIDA, FDA, DEA, Substance Abuse and Mental Health Services Administration (SAMHSA), and the 40 states with approved methadone treatment programs to make LAAM available to the patient population. Given the advantages of LAAM (i.e., it is potentially more effective therapeutically than methadone) one would conclude that narcotic treatment programs, and the states that support them, would be eager to make LAAM available to their patient populations. However, as of October 1994, fewer than 1,000 patients nationwide had received LAAM; its availability has been severely limited by laws and regulations, financing, and the approval processes (Chapter 5).

Federal Regulations

Although the federal regulations on narcotic addiction maintenance treatment (21 CFR § 291), originally included only methadone, those regulations were revised in 1989 to allow for the inclusion of other anti-addiction medications (Federal Register, 1989). In July 1993, concurrent with FDA's approval of the LAAM NDA, those treatment regulations were amended specifically to include LAAM (Federal Register, 1993). LAAM, like methadone, may be dispensed only by treatment programs approved by FDA, DEA, and designated state authorities (21 CFR § 291.505). The changes to the federal treatment regulations established a set of core standards (for such matters as patient evaluation and admission, medical and rehabilitative support services, and program sanctions) that could be applied to existing and future anti-addiction medications without requiring extensive additional rule-making. That framework preserved the opportunity to fine-tune such standards to account for the particulars of different medications (Federal Register, 1993).

In the case of LAAM, several specific restrictions on distribution were imposed to reflect the medication's characteristics as currently understood (Chapter 5). For example, the regulation prohibits take-home dosing, primarily because of LAAM's relatively lengthy time to peak effect: an uninformed patient or new user might become impatient and take illicit drugs in the interim, resulting in a potentially fatal overdose when the LAAM effect peaks [21 CFR § 291.505(k)(1)(iii); ORLAAM® package insert]. Also, the use of LAAM is prohibited in patients under 18 years of age, and strongly discouraged in pregnant women, in both cases because of an absence of relevant clinical data [21 CFR § 291.505(d)(1)(iii)(B), (d)(iv); ORLAAM® package insert].

State Regulations

In contrast to the well-coordinated regulatory effort devoted to LAAM at the federal level, the lack of coordination at the state level has seriously hampered LAAM's availability. Some of the obstacles include formulary approval and reimbursement for treatment costs (Chapter 5). The regulatory areas that pose the greatest problems, in addition to scheduling and rescheduling procedures, are the amendment of treatment regulations and the approval of treatment clinics.

Scheduling/Rescheduling

As noted above, a controlled substance such as LAAM cannot be used in treatment in a state until it has been appropriately rescheduled (or scheduled) in that state. Many variations exist from state to state, and the scheduling process can be cumbersome. For example, some states allow for automatic rescheduling based on federal rescheduling (Chapter 7), others follow a process of administrative rule-making, and many require new legislation which may take several years to enact. Additionally, some states have adopted the Uniform Controlled Substances Act, which includes a provision that directs the appropriate state officials to begin the administrative process to reschedule a controlled substance within 30 days of DEA rescheduling. However, many of the regulatory officials in those states, clearly with the authority to take action, wait for the legislature to reschedule by formal legislation. Thus, rescheduling may be a more cumbersome process than realized by simply reviewing states' laws. Finally, with regard to the rescheduling of LAAM to a Schedule II controlled substance, at least 30 states have taken action as of November 1994 (J. Thomas, BioDevelopment Corporation, personal communication).

Treatment Regulations

Each state is responsible for amending its narcotic treatment regulations to permit treatment with a new medication, such as LAAM, and for monitoring narcotic treatment programs for compliance with state regulations. As of October 1994, only 24 states had completed the procedures to include LAAM in their narcotic treatment regulations—not including California or New York (the states with 36% of the nation's narcotic treatment programs and about 45% of the opiate-dependent patient population)—where the inclusion of LAAM requires legislative action that is not expected to be completed before 1995.

Clinic Approval

Each of the estimated 650 narcotic treatment programs (which can have more than one dispensing site; in 1992 FDA licensed 737 dispensing sites) must obtain state, FDA, and DEA approvals for their programs or clinics to dispense a new drug in the treatment of opiate addiction. In the 25 states where LAAM has been included in the treatment regulations, 89 of the 302 clinics have submitted applications to FDA for clinic approval in dispensing of LAAM. As of November 1994, 52 of the 89 clinics have received state and FDA approval. Nationwide, only 7 percent of all 737 dispensing sites have received final state, FDA, and DEA approvals to dispense LAAM.

CONCLUSIONS

Each of the 50 states and the District of Columbia has the authority to regulate the research, treatment, manufacture, sale, and distribution of controlled substances through the state controlled-substances laws and treatment regulations, a situation encouraged by the federal government to prevent misuse and diversion of controlled substances. However, the lack of a uniform approach and the lack of coordination between state and federal processes regarding the development of new anti-addiction medications results in regulatory hurdles and delays. As illustrated by LAAM, regulatory regimes that were created with the intention of controlling abuse of illicit substances can prove unwieldy and counterproductive when they are applied to a therapeutic product. Of course, future anti-addiction medications might not be Schedule I or II narcotics—or even controlled substances—in which case many of the problems associated with LAAM would not occur. Inasmuch as anti-addiction medications are already perceived as a marginal business investment, the additional overlay of state laws and regulations can further deter companies from entering the field. That could be particularly true for smaller companies that have limited resources. Smaller companies may suffer an additional disadvantage if they have a limited number of products and cannot afford the time lag before realizing a return on their investment.

To be sure, potential diversion is an issue for LAAM, as it is for methadone. But the regulatory system into which LAAM has been forced takes no account of the fact that the drug was developed, in part, precisely because of specific qualities that make it less of a target for diversion than methadone. The net result is that a drug that would save money for treatment clinics and ultimately for taxpayers, that would benefit opiate-addicted patients, and that would reduce the potential for narcotic treatment products ending up in the street trade, languishes practically unused more than a year after federal approval and rescheduling.

RECOMMENDATIONS

Organizational changes are clearly needed at the state level, with federal intervention, to prevent a repeat of the LAAM case and to restore the confidence of the pharmaceutical industry that new anti-addiction medications can be developed. The committee believes that steps should be taken by federal agencies within the existing system to reduce future state regulatory obstacles. The committee proposes a two-step set of actions, interim and long-term.

Interim Actions

There are two interim steps federal agencies—the Office of National Drug
Control Policy (ONDCP), NIDA, SAMHSA, FDA, and DEA—should take under
existing authorities to ameliorate the delays, complexity, and lack of uniformity
at the state level.

**The committee recommends that federal agencies (ONDCP, NIDA,
SAMHSA, FDA, and DEA) work more closely and actively with
state regulatory authorities early in the drug development process
to prepare the path for new anti-addiction medications. That
recommendation can be implemented as follows:**

- **Identification of a regulatory point of contact in each state;**
- **Basic information could be given to the state contact early
in the drug development process (preferably no later than the submission of an NDA) about the medication, with emphasis on
characteristics that would be of most interest to state regulatory
authorities (diversion potential, target populations, or any special
characteristics that would affect how the drug would be dispensed,
such as dosing frequency). To the extent that any of the information
is proprietary and confidential, the developer's permission for such
disclosure would have to be obtained.**
- **As the medication moves closer to FDA approval, federal
agencies could ensure that the necessary state regulatory processes
begin immediately after approval, or, if state regulations permit,
even before—such as upon the issuance of an approvable letter.**
- **Federal agencies could work with the state contact, as the
product moves through the state regulatory process, to correct any
problems as they arise.**

**The committee recommends that ONDCP, in cooperation with FDA,
DEA, SAMHSA, and NIDA, take an active role in compiling
relevant information about state regulatory processes for anti-
addiction medications that are categorized as narcotics and educating state regulators and pharmaceutical company representatives
about the processes and their practical consequences. To implement
that recommendation, the following steps may be taken:**

- **Conduct a comprehensive study of state laws and regulations pertinent to the development of anti-addiction medications
that are controlled substances, and develop a step-by-step manual**

for pharmaceutical companies explaining the mechanisms involved in launching an anti-addiction medication.

•   Establish and maintain on-line access to the comprehensive study, as well as to state regulatory information of a practical nature (for example, a directory of relevant state officials) to facilitate pharmaceutical company access.

•   Sponsor nationwide or regional educational meetings for state authorities and clinic administrators to disseminate information about potential anti-addiction medications.

Long-Term Actions

Ultimately, close attention should be given to reforming the current patchwork of state regulations. The committee considered complete federal preemption of state controlled-substance laws and regulations insofar as those authorities affect the development of anti-addiction medications, but it concluded that such a proposal would go beyond what is strictly necessary and could be politically unrealistic. The committee does believe, however, that the initiative for reform must come from the federal government, and that it must involve some form of legislative change.

The committee recommends, on the basis of the comprehensive study recommended above, that ONDCP, in coordination with other relevant federal agencies, develop a series of specific actions encouraging states to reform their laws and regulations to facilitate the availability of new anti-addiction medications that are controlled substances.[2] Those actions should give particular attention to:

•   **Modifying state laws and regulations for narcotic treatment programs to remove the need to reopen and amend the laws or regulations to accommodate each new product.**
•   **Imposing specific deadlines for state regulatory action in response to FDA approval of a new anti-addiction medication that requires state action to be dispensed to patients.**

---

[2]ONDCP has previously drafted and put forth model state legislation on numerous topics, thus there is a precedent for model legislation on research and development of anti-addiction medications.

- Developing flexible, alternative means of controlling the dispensing of anti-addiction narcotic medications that would avoid the "methadone model" of individually approved treatment centers.

Finally, the committee urges that Congress, in cooperation with the National Conference of Commissioners on Uniform State Laws, draft legislation requiring states to implement needed changes, rather than preempt outright the relevant state laws or regulations. The legislation could establish regulatory benchmarks (such as the length of time allowed after FDA approval for the state to take legislative or other action; types of alternative dispensing controls). That legislation could be freestanding or as an amendment to NATA.

Clearly, if the federal government wishes to remove regulatory obstacles to the development of anti-addiction medications, significant changes in current policies, laws, and regulations are necessary.

REFERENCES

Federal Register. 1989. Food and Drug Administration, National Institute on Drug Abuse, Methadone in Maintenance and Detoxification; Joint Revision of Conditions for Use (final rule). 54: 8954.

Federal Register. 1993. Food and Drug Administration, Levo-Alpha-Acetylmethadol (LAAM) in Maintenance: Revision of Conditions for Use in the Treatment of Narcotic Addiction (LAAM Interim Rule). 58: 38,704.

Massachusetts Bureau of Substance Abuse Services. No date given. Outpatient Methadone Services: Primary Service Elements and Staffing Requirements Attachment.

NCJA (National Criminal Justice Association). 1991. Guide to State Controlled Substances Acts. Washington, DC: NCJA.

Research Advisory Panel. 1993. 24th Annual Report of the Research Advisory Panel, State of California. San Francisco: Research Advisory Panel.

SAMHSA (Substance Abuse and Mental Health Services Administration). 1992. Approval and Monitoring of Narcotic Treatment Programs: A Guide on the Roles of Federal and State Agencies. Rockville, MD: SAMHSA.

9

Market Obstacles and Creating Incentives

The disincentives to the pharmaceutical industry for the development of anti-addiction medications are formidable (Figure 9.1). The paucity of pharmacotherapies for the treatment of drug dependence illustrates the point. Despite the recognized success of methadone and the promise of a longer-acting agent, levo-alpha-acetylmethadol (LAAM), in the treatment of opiate addiction, there have been no novel anti-opiate medications developed for 30 years,[1] and there is no medication specifically for the treatment of cocaine addiction. That this lack of success persists, despite the dire health, social, and economic consequences of drug addiction, further attests to the many barriers faced by the pharmaceutical industry. The committee believes, however, that many of the barriers can be overcome with changes in government policies and a full commitment of resources to this area of medications development.

The committee aware of the disincentives to industry, yet cognizant of the need for pharmacotherapies, grappled with the issue of presenting extraordinary incentives to the pharmaceutical industry. Many of the issues and ideas were presented at the June 13, 1994, IOM workshop (Appendix F) by industry representatives and other concerned individuals and were discussed at great length by the committee. These include granting a patent extension on some other product marketed by a pharmaceutical company that developed an anti-addiction medication, removing the potential for price controls, allowing advance

---

[1]With the exception of naltrexone, approved in 1984, for the treatment of opiate addiction.

special purchase of anti-addiction medications, and/or creating a prize or bounty to the first few companies that produce an approved anti-addiction medication. The committee could not adequately envision the implementation of those extraordinary incentives, and they are not presented as committee recommendations. However, a majority of the committee agreed that some of the incentives regarded as extraordinary should be deliberated by policy makers. Those issues that had majority support from committee members are presented later in the chapter, not as recommendations but as approaches for further consideration.

A fundamental tenet of this report is that innovative pharmacotherapies for the treatment of drug addiction are most likely to be developed through an effective public-private sector partnership involving the National Institute on Drug Abuse (NIDA) and a limited number of committed pharmaceutical or biotechnology companies. That approach has been applied successfully by several of the National Institutes of Health (NIH) institutes to stimulate the development of new drugs, for example, in the fields of cancer, acquired immune deficiency syndrome (AIDS), and epilepsy (Appendix E); the Medications Development Division of NIDA was established to accomplish the same objective for drug dependence (Chapter 3). However, a variety of reasons, including limited scientific understanding of the physiological bases of addiction, craving, and relapse, numerous marketing obstacles, and the failure to identify pharmacotherapeutic research and pharmacotherapies as national priorities, have prevented NIDA from forming effective partnerships.

The committee notes that any progress in attracting the private sector to the difficult task of developing new anti-addiction medications will require strong and sustained federal leadership and research support. Strong leadership is needed at the highest levels of the federal government to foster an environment that supports the treatment of drug dependence. The effectiveness and cost-effectiveness of pharmacotherapies need to be clearly articulated to the public, to involved government agencies, to the academic and treatment communities, and to industry. Sustained support for basic research in neuropharmacology (specifically the physiological bases of addiction, craving, and relapse) and continued support for clinical research by the executive branch and the Congress must be a priority.

The committee believes that, at a minimum, strong federal leadership and research support are essential for progress to be made in attracting private-sector research and development in the area of anti-addiction medications. Without support for those two areas, incentives, no matter how attractive, will not be sufficient to attract the industry to this field of medications development.

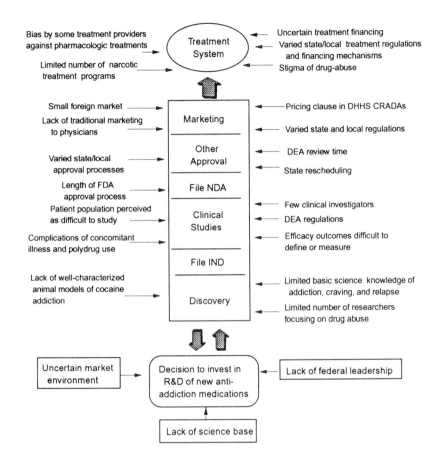

FIGURE 9.1 Current problems in the development of anti-addiction medications.

MARKET OBSTACLES TO PRIVATE-SECTOR INVESTMENT

To further identify the barriers to private-sector investment for the development and marketing of anti-addiction medications and to formulate viable policy options as possible solutions, the committee sought the opinions and suggestions of pharmaceutical industry executives, the scientific community, and federal and state government agency representatives (Appendix A). The committee conducted a survey of pharmaceutical companies (Appendix D), met with the Institute of Medicine (IOM) Forum on Drug Development, and held a Workshop on Policies to Stimulate Private Sector Development of Anti-Addiction Medications (Appendix F); which focused on marketing, regulatory, research and training, and treatment-financing issues.

New products are developed by pharmaceutical companies for many reasons, the most important of which is to increase company sales in existing and new markets (Spilker, 1989). Companies must examine many factors, including those listed below, and calculate the probabilities of an adequate return on their investment before deciding to enter a new area of drug development (Spilker, 1989). In the field of developing anti-addiction medications, the overwhelming majority of the following factors are problematic.

- the size of the market;
- the cost of developing and marketing a drug;
- the price of the drug;
- the length of time the drug will be protected with a patent;
- the social attitudes about the drug;
- the regulatory requirements for development and approval;
- the time required to develop the drug;
- clinical feasibility;
- medical value;
- commercial value;
- probability of achieving marketing success;
- legal considerations; and
- competitive value.

Many of those issues have been discussed in the report, the remainder are discussed below.

Nature and Size of the Market

From the pharmaceutical industry's point of view the size of the potential market for determining investment in research and development (R&D), is not estimated simply from the absolute number of patients with a given condition.

For example, there are about 2.1 million cocaine-dependent individuals and 500,000 to 1 million opiate-dependent individuals in the United States (Hunt and Rhodes, 1992; Kreek, 1992). Those numbers are high enough to be attractive from a marketing perspective, yet there is significantly more pharmaceutical activity in other areas with comparable or much smaller patient populations. Approximately 25,000 individuals have amyotrophic lateral sclerosis (ALS or Lou Gehrig's disease), for which several pharmaceutical companies have compounds in various stages of clinical development (Samotin, 1994). Similarly, the market for medications to treat the 2.1 million epilepsy patients is well established at $400 million to $500 million, and three new products have been or are about to be approved (Samotin, 1994). The pharmaceutical industry appears willing to invest in R&D for markets that are smaller in size or approximately the same size as the number of cocaine-dependent individuals, yet reluctant to enter the field of anti-addiction products. There are several reasons for this apparent paradox.

First, there is a perceived lack of a market, by the pharmaceutical industry, in terms of true medical demand, access to patients, and motivation of patients. It is believed that a portion of the population is either not interested in treatment or erratic in compliance. Second, one segment of treatment providers is committed to a "drug-free" concept. Third, any particular medication is likely to be useful for a particular indication (such as reducing the craving for cocaine) and not for treating the entire drug-dependent population. The result is greater uncertainty in predicting the demand or true market size for new anti-addiction medications than for drugs intended for more established markets (Samotin, 1994). However, those niches represent opportunities, especially for small pharmaceutical companies, biotechnology companies, and those already involved in the development of central nervous system (CNS) compounds, that have not been fully explored by the industry. Furthermore, an uncharted market coupled with the limits in the basic science of addiction (Chapter 2) present a significant obstacle in the discovery and delivery of anti-addiction medications.

For pharmaceutical companies making decisions about new areas for R&D, the factor of market size is interwoven with the issues of the costs of developing and marketing a new medication, pricing, and reimbursement because those factors determine the financial return on sales. To address the issue of return on investment, the committee has endorsed a host of recommendations throughout the report for the federal government to consider and offers additional recommendations in this chapter to offset the major obstacles.

The Orphan Drug Act (Public Law 97-414) was enacted to stimulate the market in the development of medications for rare diseases by granting market exclusivity to companies who developed those compounds (Chapter 7). The standard for orphan status is whether a drug is intended to treat a disease or condition that affects fewer than 200,000 persons in the United States or that affects more than 200,000 but for which there is no reasonable expectation of recovering development costs from sales in the United States. Since the passage of the Orphan Drug Act in 1983, the pharmaceutical industry has marketed 60 medications for orphan diseases, and the Food and Drug Administration (FDA) has granted 488 orphan drug designations (Sanders, 1993). The Orphan Drug Act similarly could be used as a mechanism to provide market exclusivity to companies with FDA approved anti-addiction medications. The committee believes that the FDA should consider the actual patient population likely to be treated, rather than those potentially treatable, as there is probably a large segment of the drug-dependent population that will never present for pharmacotherapy. It is illogical and counterproductive to the purposes of the Orphan Drug Act to count those patients against the 200,000 threshold.

The committee recommends that FDA interpret the Orphan Drug Act broadly with the intent of granting orphan drug status to FDA-approved anti-addiction medications whose potential market can reasonably be judged to meet the 200,000 patient criterion stipulated by law. Alternatively, new legislation similar to the Orphan Drug Act could be drafted specifically for FDA-approved anti-addiction medications.

This is a more explicit recommendation than the one previously stated in the committee's preliminary report issued March 1994.[2] The committee believes that the designation of orphan or orphanlike status for approved anti-addiction medications is necessary to stimulate market investment as financial return is limited, given the nature of the anti-addiction market.

Drug Pricing and Intellectual Property Rights

In 1986, Congress passed the Federal Technology and Transfer Act (P.L. 99-502) to encourage private companies to commercialize federal inventions. The statute authorizes federal laboratories to enter into cooperative research and development agreements (CRADAs) with nonprofit institutions and private companies. CRADAs enable government agencies to negotiate exclusive commercialization licenses with industry partners. In 1989, NIH made an

---

[2]The March 1994 recommendation read as follows. "The committee recommends that further exploration of the possibility of special incentives similar to the Orphan Drug Act or other legislation for anti-addiction medications be considered."

administrative decision to adopt a reasonable (or fair) pricing clause[3] into its CRADAs in response to complaints about the introductory price of AZT (zidovudine), an AIDS medication, which was deemed excessive at $10,000 per patient per year. AZT was developed through a cooperative agreement. Such pricing provisions are included in NIH exclusive licensing agreements.

The potential effect of CRADAs on pricing of products and on patent rights has been an important issue of concern for the pharmaceutical industry. Industry representatives have noted that the "reasonable pricing clause" is an important deterrent to a long-term, effective partnership between the government and the private sector. It views the provisions as too broad and too threatening to proprietary interests (Chapter 3; U.S. DHHS, 1993).

The committee also heard from industry that the CRADA process is lengthy and complex, often taking about a year for final approval and requiring many layers of review. Industry officials noted their frustration with the process required to establish a CRADA, which, rather than encourage innovative research, acts as another disincentive. NIH is fully aware of the controversy, and is currently reassessing its CRADA policy. There have been two public meetings (July 21 and September 8, 1994) on the issue.

Inasmuch as the language of the reasonable pricing clause was adopted by administrative action within NIH, it is not required by law, and NIH could resolve the controversy by administrative action and at the same time protect the interests of the public.

The committee recommends that administrative action be taken by NIH to resolve the issue of reasonable pricing in CRADAs. However, if NIH is unsuccessful in stimulating the industry to form cooperative agreements, then the committee recommends legislative action to remove or modify the reasonable pricing clause.[4]

In the absence of a definition of a "fair or reasonable price" and in light of NIH's lack of expertise to undertake meaningful analyses of private-sector pricing decisions (OTA, 1993; U.S. DHHS, 1993), the committee believes that

---

[3]Section 8.3 of the NIH Patent Policy Board's Model CRADA states that the institutes' concern is that "there be a reasonable relationship between the pricing of a licensed product, the public investment in that product, and the health and safety needs of the public. Accordingly, exclusive commercialization licenses granted for NIH intellectual property rights may require that this relationship be supported by reasonable evidence."

[4]This recommendation is revised from the committee's preliminary report published in March 1994.

this obstacle should be removed. Additionally, NIH should take steps to streamline the CRADA process. NIH could assign additional staff members or establish a centralized committee to eliminate the need for multiple levels of review and provide a single site for negotiating and approving CRADAs (IOM Workshop, June 13, 1994).

Societal Stigma

The societal stigma of developing and marketing a medication for treating drug-dependent patients is a concern for pharmaceutical companies. They fear that, once a medication is approved for use in the treatment of drug addiction, the market for other indications will diminish or disappear. Eli Lilly's experience with methadone illustrates the point. Methadone was developed as an analgesic, but its use for pain relief significantly diminished once it became widely used as a treatment for heroin addiction. Patients, in general, do not want to take a medication associated with drug addiction. Thus, the pharmaceutical industry is understandably reluctant to develop compounds specifically for drug addiction, if other medical uses for the compounds are possible.

There is no easy solution to the problem of stigma associated with drug addiction and its treatment. However, the committee stresses the need for national leadership in support of pharmacotherapy and continued emphasis on prevention and treatment. The sense of stigma is most likely to diminish as a result of public education and broader acceptance of addiction as a treatable disease.

Clinical Research on Anti-Addiction Medications

Clinical research in the drug-addicted population is inherently difficult. There are numerous problems in setting up clinical trials for drug-addicted patients, for example, there are relatively few experienced investigators (Chapter 6), patients are commonly unreliable and follow-up difficult, efficacy end points may be difficult to define or measure, safety evaluation is confounded by adverse events due to such concomitant illnesses as tuberculosis (TB) and AIDS, and studies can be difficult to control appropriately or to conduct on a blinded basis. In addition, if the drug under evaluation is a controlled substance, the regulatory requirements of the Drug Enforcement Administration (DEA) and of each state's narcotics-control agency must be met (Chapters 7 and 8). This daunting set of scientific and procedural barriers has discouraged most pharmaceutical companies from considering clinical studies in this field (Mossinghoff, 1989).

One of the major accomplishments of the Medications Development Division (MDD) in developing LAAM, as described in Chapter 3, was to cope successfully with those barriers. MDD organized successful multicenter clinical trials that included expedited FDA drug approval. In this accomplishment, MDD not only completed the development of LAAM but organized a network of clinics and investigators that could participate in future Phase III studies of other drugs. Such a network could be complemented by the existence of national drug-abuse research centers (Chapters 2 and 6). Those centers could provide additional scientific expertise and facilities for conducting clinical research in clinical pharmacology and early efficacy studies on promising new drugs for the treatment of addiction.

The pharmaceutical executives who met with the committee indicated that the centers (as proposed) plus a network of investigators, for Phase III studies, would be of great value in overcoming one of the important disincentives to the private sector in this field. Equally important, from their point of view, is the effective working relationship established between MDD and FDA, as a result of the LAAM experience. They emphasized that an MDD function of "honest broker" or "dispassionate scientific adviser" both to companies developing new drugs under investigational new drug applications (INDs) and to the FDA would be welcomed. The NIDA and FDA officials who met with the committee felt similarly, but they were concerned that resource constraints in the future might limit their ability to devote adequate attention to this function. The committee believes, however, that NIDA and FDA must continue to build on this relationship of trust, and it urges a formalization of the relationship between NIDA and FDA.

The committee recommends a memorandum of understanding signed by both the director of NIH and the commissioner of FDA that would detail publicly the working relationship between NIDA and FDA.

This relationship is an important long-term asset to both agencies. It can serve as the basis for continuing communication and productive effort in the development of anti-addiction medications while maintaining the scientific independence of NIDA and the regulatory role of FDA.

Product Liability

Product liability and the risk of lawsuits, as a result of unforeseen patient injury, are often cited by the industry as major uncertainties in the marketing of a new drug. In the case of drugs for addiction, especially for opiate and cocaine addiction, this risk is thought to be particularly high in precisely the patients who, from a public-health standpoint, would need treatment the most, e.g., drug users who are pregnant, infected with human immunodeficiency virus (HIV) and/or infected with TB (Mossinghoff, 1989).

Industry representatives pointed out that they are not aware of any drugs specifically approved by FDA for the treatment of associated illness in pregnant patients or labeled as safe for use in pregnancy (pregnancy category A in the package insert); this was confirmed by FDA officials (R. Temple, personal communication). The reluctance to seek such approval stems largely from experience with Bendectin, a drug once marketed for nausea and vomiting of pregnancy that was withdrawn from the market by its manufacturer because of protracted litigation over a large number of product-liability lawsuits that alleged birth defects in spite of epidemiological evidence and failure of FDA reviews to confirm such toxicity (Sheffield and Batagol, 1985). The lesson, as far as individual drug manufacturers are concerned, is that they cannot afford to market a drug specifically labeled for use in pregnancy. However, as the committee pursued this issue as an obstacle for the development of anti-addiction medications, they discovered that it is of general concern for pharmaceutical companies and not isolated to the development of anti-addiction medications.

NEED FOR FEDERAL LEADERSHIP

The committee has considered and attempted to bring clarity to the multiple components involved in the development of anti-addiction medications. Such development depends critically on cooperation between the public and private sectors. Yet the number of federal agencies involved, current agency funding and staffing levels, regulatory requirements, remaining scientific questions, and other issues present difficult challenges to successful partnership and cooperation. Although many of the challenges are addressed in this report, it is important to recognize that government policies have not provided a strong emphasis on pharmacotherapy for the treatment of drug addiction. This lack of federal leadership represents an additional disincentive to industry, in that it affects the public sector's ability to establish clear guidelines, enhance interagency cooperation, and provide research programs with the stability necessary for medication discovery and development. In addition to its role in developing medications for drug addiction, the government is likely to be the major purchaser of those medications. Thus, government policies are critical in determining the environment in which such medications are developed and are necessary for supporting pharmacotherapy as an important and accepted form of treatment.

The committee applauds the current emphasis on treatment in the 1994 National Drug Control Strategy and suggests an additional action to underscore the importance of treatment and strengthen federal leadership.

One option might be for the President to issue an executive order assigning a high priority to the development of medications for drug-abuse treatment. This, or some other explicit action, would enhance cooperation among the government agencies involved, focus their activities, and aid in the removal of existing institutional barriers.

Explicit action at the Presidential or cabinet level would have the added benefit of signaling to the private sector that the development of anti-addiction medications is a matter of high national priority. The committee further believes that progress in this area should be monitored. Thus, any action taken should include a provision for reporting by the involved agencies regarding their efforts to coordinate with other agencies and remove barriers identified. Examples of specific ways in which cooperation could expedite development of anti-addiction medications are formalization of agreements between NIDA and the Department of Veterans Affairs (DVA) for support of clinical trials, and encouragement of all agencies to promote cooperation with the private sector. Other strategies, including the use of executive-level task forces and commissions, may also be options to strengthen federal leadership and give the issue high priority in the eyes of both the public and private sectors.

CONCLUSIONS

In reviewing the obstacles presented to the pharmaceutical industry (Figure 9.1) for the development of anti-addiction medications, it is clear that, the disincentives outweigh the incentives. The formidable scientific and marketing issues, regulatory complexities, and financial uncertainties add up to an unattractive picture to the pharmaceutical industry, which tends to enter R&D investment from a high risk-high reward perspective.

Although it is possible to envision incentives that would interest some pharmaceutical companies (e.g., small pharmaceutical companies, biotechnology companies, or those companies already involved in the development of CNS compounds) without strong federal leadership, in establishing the role of pharmacotherapy and a long-term federal commitment to research, the committee believes all other efforts are likely to falter. As the federal government considers policies that will remove obstacles, the committee suggests a tiered approach of incentives, allowing each tier of incentives time to produce the desired effect. For example, the first action may be the removal of disincentives, then the creation of modest incentives, and finally the development of extraordinary incentives.

The removal of disincentives includes many of the committee's administrative recommendations: use of orphan drug and fast track mechanisms for anti-addiction compounds; removal of adverse effects on clinical research of Drug Enforcement Administration (DEA) requirements under the Controlled Substances Act; and counting DEA review time as part of the regulatory process for purposes of patent term extension for controlled substances.

The creation of modest incentives should include broad interpretation of the Orphan Drug Act to include anti-addiction medications or similar legislation to stimulate the market in the development of anti-addiction medications; a strong federal leadership role in support of treatment of drug-dependent patients; funding of basic research and training; adequate funding of treatment; and a modification or elimination of the "reasonable pricing clause" in CRADAs.

Finally, the committee considered two extraordinary incentives that the executive branch and the Congress may wish to consider. They are presented below as options for consideration, and they are not committee recommendations.

OPTIONS FOR FURTHER CONSIDERATION

The committee discussed whether the overall strategy (i.e., strong federal leadership regarding drug abuse treatment and support of research) coupled with removal of obstacles to anti-addiction medication R&D would be likely to result in activity by the pharmaceutical industry. Additionally, the committee considered whether a considerable economic incentive specifically intended to reward the development of new anti-addiction medications was needed. The Committee did not reach a consensus on that issue and has no formal recommendation for such an extraordinary incentive.

Nevertheless, the Committee wishes to include in this report a brief description of two incentives that were supported by a majority of its members, recognizing that the committee has not provided details for implementation of those incentives. Both of the following proposals are limited to medications developed for cocaine addiction and are intended to create a guaranteed market in view of the limited potential for return on investment of anti-addiction medications as perceived by the pharmaceutical industry.

Option 1 would offer developers of the first few (e.g., two or three) FDA-approved medications for the treatment of cocaine addiction for 3 years after approval a federal subsidy of a maximum of $50 million for purchase of the drug. The subsidy could be given, for example, through reimbursement of the copayment portion of medications for patients with health insurance and the full cost of medications for those patients without medical insurance.

Option 2 would allow for standing federal purchase orders for prearranged quantities and at an adequate price of one or more new cocaine treatment medications to begin at the time of FDA approval. The purchase orders would establish unambiguous confirmation of a market demand for those products, thereby stimulating investment and commercialization.

The options presented above were favored by a majority of the committee. Most committee members also favored implementation of those extraordinary incentives only if the first two tiers of recommendations fail to stimulate progress in the anti-addiction medications market. A majority of the committee agreed, however, that the above options should be deliberated by the executive branch and Congress as they develop policies to stimulate this area of research and development.

REFERENCES

Hunt DE, Rhodes W. 1992. Characteristics of Heavy Cocaine Users Including Polydrug Use, Criminal Activity, and Health Risks. Prepared for the Office of National Drug Control Policy by Abt Associates, Inc.

Kreek MJ. 1992. Rationale for maintenance pharmacotherapy of opiate dependence. In: O'Brien CP, Jaffe JH, eds. Addictive States. New York: Raven Press. 205–230.

Mossinghoff GJ. 1989. Letter to Senator Joseph R. Biden, Jr. re: PMA survey of research and development programs in the development of treatments for drug addiction. December 1, 1989.

OTA (Office of Technology Assessment). 1993. Pharmaceutical R&D: Costs, Risks and Rewards. Washington, DC: Government Printing Office. OTA-H-522.

Samotin S. 1994. Size of the Cocaine Market. Presentation to the IOM Workshop on Policies to Stimulate Private Sector Development of Anti-Addiction Medications. June 13, 1994. Washington, DC. National Academy of Sciences.

Sanders CA. 1993. The Orphan Drug Act: should it be changed? Archives of Internal Medicine 153:2623–2625.

Sheffield LJ, Batagol R. 1985. The creation of therapeutic orphans—or, what have we learnt from the Debendox fiasco? Medical Journal of Australia 143:143–7.

Spilker B. 1989. Multinational Drug Companies: Issues in Drug Discovery and Development. New York: Raven Press.

U.S. DHHS (U.S. Department of Health and Human Services), Office of Inspector General. 1993. Technology Transfer and the Public Interest: Cooperative Research and Development Agreements at NIH. OEI-01-92-01100.

Appendix A

Acknowledgments

The committee would like to thank the following persons who shared their expertise.

John Abbott
National Institute on Drug Abuse

John Ambre
American Medical Association

Robert Angarola
Hyman, Phelps and McNamara

Douglas Anglin
University of California

Bruce Artim
National Institutes of Health

Dennis Baker
Texas Department of Health

John F. Beary
Pharmaceutical Research and
  Manufacturers of America

Martin Becker, Esq.
New York, NY

Walter Bell
National Institute of Neurological
  Disorders and Stroke

Leslie Benet
University of California

Shawn Bentley
Senate Judiciary Committee

Alex Bradford
BioDevelopment Corporation

Peter Bridge
National Institute on Drug Abuse

Bruce Burlington
Food and Drug Administration

William Butynski
National Association of State
  Alcohol and Drug Abuse
  Directors

Robert Callahan
American Society of
  Addiction Medicine, Inc.

Neal Castagnoli
Virginia State University

John Coleman
Drug Enforcement
  Administration

Shirley Coletti
McCormick Research Center

Joseph Collins
Department of Veterans Affairs

Tim Condon
National Institute on Drug Abuse

Gary Coody
Texas Department of Health

James Cooper
National Institute on Drug Abuse

Addie Corradi
New York State Office of
  Alcoholism and Substance
  Abuse Services

Paul Coulis
National Institute on Drug Abuse

Lee Cummings
National Institute on Drug Abuse

Albert Derivan
Wyeth-Ayerst Research

George DeVaux
BioDevelopment Corporation

Kay Dickersin
University of Maryland
  School of Medicine

Carl W. Dieffenbach
National Institute of Allergy
  and Infectious Diseases

Herman Diesenhaus
Substance Abuse and Mental
  Health Services Administration

Christopher Doherty
Fox, Bennett and Turner

Jack Durell
Treatment Research Institute

Robert Eaton
Pharmaceutical Manufacturers
  Association

Barbara Espey
Massachusetts Department of
  Public Health

Susan Everingham
RAND

Rachel Feldman
Lewin-VHI, Inc.

Marian Fischman
Columbia University

Michael Friedman
National Cancer Institute

Judy Galloway
Substance Abuse and Mental
  Health Services Administration

Fred Garcia
Office of National Drug
  Control Policy

Ronald Garity
Medco Behavioral Care

Ann Geller
American Society of
  Addiction Medicine

Dee Gillespie
DuPont Pharmaceutical

Thomas Gitchel
Drug Enforcement
  Administration

Richard Golden
Department of Alcohol and Drug
  Programs, State of California

Avram Goldstein
Stanford University

Frederick K. Goodwin
National Institute of
  Mental Health

Eric Goplerud
Substance Abuse and Mental
  Health Services Administration

John Gregrich
Office of National Drug
  Control Policy

Steve Grossman
Hill and Knowlton

Charles Grudzinskas
National Institute on Drug Abuse

Gene Haislip
Drug Enforcement
  Administration

Louis Harris
Medical College of Virginia

Christine Hartel
National Institute on Drug Abuse

Henrick Harwood
Lewin-VHI, Inc.

Richard Hawks
National Institute on Drug Abuse

Rebecca Henderson
Massachusetts Institute of
  Technology

Carol Hubner
National Institute on Drug Abuse

James Isbister
Pharmavene, Inc.

David Joranson
University of Wisconsin
  Medical School

Ruth Kahn
Health Resources and Services
Administration

Janice F. Kauffman
Substance Abuse Treatment
Services

Tom Kellenberger
Medco Containment Services

Richard Kilburg
Johns Hopkins University

Richard Kitz
Massachusetts General Hospital

Delbert Konnor
American Managed Care
Pharmacy Association

Thomas Kosten
Yale University

Harvey Kupferberg
National Institute of Neurological
Disorders and Stroke

Laurie Kurtzman
New York State Office
of Alcoholism and
Drug Abuse Services

Irwin Lerner
Hoffmann-La Roche

Robert Levy
Wyeth-Ayerst Research

David Lewis
Brown University

Robert Lubran
Substance Abuse and Mental
Health Services Administration

Karen Marquis
Wyeth-Ayerst

David W. Martin, Jr.
Du Pont Merck
Pharmaceutical Company

David McCann
National Institute on Drug Abuse

Mary Elizabeth McCaul
Johns Hopkins University
Hospital

Howard McClain
Drug Enforcement
Administration

Catherine McCormack
Generic Pharmaceutical
Industry Association

Thomas McLellan
Penn-VA Center for Studies
of Addiction

Daniel Melnick
Substance Abuse and Mental
Health Services Administration

Richard Merrill
University of Virginia
School of Law

Harry Meyer
American Cyanamid Company

Corrine Moody
Food and Drug Administration

Ed Morgan
Substance Abuse and Mental
  Health Services Administration

Dave Neuenschwander
Mallinckrodt Chemical, Inc.

Stuart Nightingale
Food and Drug Administration

Stanley Novick
National Alliance of Methadone
  Advocates

John A. Oates
Vanderbilt University

Mark Parrino
American Methadone Treatment
  Association

Nancy Payte
Drug Dependence Associates

Thomas Payte
Drug Dependence Associates

Dana Peale
Cure is Not Worse

Chris Putala
Senate Judiciary Committee

Scott Reines
Merck Research Laboratories

Nicholas P. Reuter
Food and Drug Administration

Peter Riddell
RAND

Barbara Roberts
Office of National Drug
  Control Policy

Sheri L. Samotin
The Wilkerson Group, Inc.

Charles Sanders
Glaxo Inc.

Frank Sapienza
Drug Enforcement
  Administration

Alan Sartorelli
Yale University
  School of Medicine

Clifford Scharke
National Institutes of Health

Saul Schepartz
National Cancer Institute

David Schieser
California Research
  Advisory Panel

Sam Schildhaus
Office of National Drug
  Control Policy

Ian Shaffer
Value Behavioral Health

Dale Shoemaker
National Cancer Institute

Robert Sisko
International Coalition
  for Addict Self Help

Eve Slater
Merck Research Laboratory

Michael Smith
Lincoln Hospital, New York

Marvin Snyder
National Institute on Drug Abuse

Solomon Snyder
Johns Hopkins University

Steve Tabscot
Texas Methadone Provider
  Group

Robert Temple
Food and Drug Administration

John Thomas
BioDevelopment Corporation

Richard Thoreson
Substance Abuse and Mental
  Health Services Administration

Alan Trachtenberg
National Institute on Drug Abuse

Frank Vocci
National Institute on Drug Abuse

Jeane Van Lear
Biotechnology Industry
  Organization

William Vodra
Arnold and Porter

Ellen Weber
Legal Action Center

Bonnie Wilford
George Washington University

Curtis Wright
Food and Drug Administration

Paul Wohlford
Substance Abuse and Mental
  Health Services Administration

Thomas Wyatt
National Association of
  State Controlled Substance
  Authorities

Michael Young
Proctor & Gamble

Appendix B

Organization and Mission Statements of NIDA's Medications Development Division and Its Branches

MEDICATIONS DEVELOPMENT DIVISION
MISSION STATEMENT

(1) Plans and directs studies necessary to identify, evaluate, develop and obtain FDA marketing approval for new medications for the treatment of drug dependence and addiction and other brain and behavioral disorders; (2) develops and administers a national program of basic and clinical pharmaceutical research to develop innovative biological and pharmacological treatment approaches; (3) supports training in the fundamental sciences and clinical disciplines related to the pharmacotherapeutic treatment of drug abuse; (4) collaborates with: (a) the pharmaceutical and chemical industry in the United States and other Nations and, (b) the Federal medications development programs; and (5) works closely with FDA in assuring that research designed to show the clinical efficacy of new compounds is evaluated and approved in the most expeditious manner possible.

Biometrics Branch Mission Statement

(1) Provides consultation and advice on study design and analysis issues involved in pharmacology, toxicology, pharmacokinetics, and clinical trials for intramural and extramural projects of interest to the Division; (2) provides consultation on design and analysis issues regarding medications being developed by the pharmaceutical industry for clinical indications subsumed under the Division's responsibilities; and (3) analyzes preclinical and clinical data for medications development projects, using established methodologies as appropriate

and developing new analysis methods when current methods are judged inappropriate.

Chemistry and Pharmaceutics Branch Mission Statement

(1) Administers a national program of research and development in the following areas: (a) medicinal and synthetic chemistry, and discovery of new chemicals of therapeutic value; (b) bioavailability, pharmacokinetics and drug metabolism studies and studies on the interactions of these compounds with known drugs of abuse, including fetal exposure; and (c) bulk chemical preparation and dosage form preparation of medications under development carried out in compliance with the FDA Good Manufacturing Practice regulations; (2) develops and manages: (a) an SAR database for data on compounds of interest to the Medications Development Division; and (b) new rapid screening projects which generate pharmacological activity and storage of such data in a computer database and coordination of screening programs with other sources of data of potential interest to the Division; (3) provides analytical chemistry development and services including development of assay methods for applications of drug characterization, bioavailability and kinetic studies in the Division, and centralized analysis of biological specimens (e.g., urine for cocaine use detection); (4) manages the distribution of controlled substances and related compounds, research chemicals, bulk pharmaceuticals, dosage forms which are used in programs associated with medications development; (5) provides documentation of testing of new drug substances and dosage forms for Investigational New Drug application and New Drug Application reports for drugs developed in the Division; and (6) provides consultation and technical support for urine testing of drugs of abuse in clinical trials being conducted for the Division.

Clinical Trials Branch Mission Statement

(1) Plans, designs, and implements a comprehensive program of extramural clinical studies, in coordination with intramural projects, evaluating new and marketed drugs for their potential value in treating substance abuse disorders; (2) provides consultation to the other ADAMHA Institutes regarding medications development, patient recruitment, investigator and site selection, and other administrative clinical issues; (3) files Investigation New Drug applications for clinical projects in conjunction with the Regulatory Affairs Branch; (4) designs and monitors clinical trials for safety and efficacy of new and currently marketed drugs in the treatment of substance abuse disorders;

(5) provides consultation and collaboration with the pharmaceutical industry regarding projects of mutual interest; and (6) supports research training of clinicians to increase the skills, quantity, quality, and utilization of research in medications development.

Pharmacology and Toxicology Branch Mission Statement

(1) Plans, designs, implements, and coordinates a comprehensive program of extramural studies, in coordination with intramural projects, evaluating the efficacy of potential medications in preclinical pharmacological models; (2) plans, designs, and implements a comprehensive program of preclinical toxicological studies conducted under Good Laboratory Practices regulations for the purpose of determining the safety of potential medications; (3) evaluates the interactive effects of potential medications with drugs of abuse in preclinical models; (4) recommends compounds for further testing in animal models and coordinated testing of compounds under development with the other branches of the Division; (5) recommends compounds for human testing for potential efficacy in substance abuse disorders; (6) develops data storage capacities for preclinical pharmacological and toxicological data; and (7) provides liaison, consultation, and collaboration with the Food and Drug Administration and the pharmaceutical industry on matters related to preclinical models of drug abuse and drug dependence.

Regulatory Affairs Branch Mission Statement

(1) Provides legal and regulatory advice and support to the Division's medication development activities; (2) coordinates the Division's activities in technology transfer and development, including the development and negotiation of Cooperative Research and Development Agreements, Material Transfer Agreements, interagency agreements and contracts; (3) maintains liaison with the Office of the General Counsel, Office of the Secretary, the Patent Branch of the Office of General Counsel,NIH and the Office of Technology Transfer, NIH; (4) maintains liaison with the Food and Drug Administration, and files Investigational New Drug applications and New Drug Applications as necessary; (5) develops and maintains a management information database and library functions, assuring that proprietary and confidential information are appropriately safeguarded; (6) serves as project managers coordinating a variety of patent, regulatory, business and data functions, including electronic filing and storage of data, marketing surveys, access to consultants and new systems to keep the program current;

(7) provides briefings, reports, and congressional testimony as required; and (8) serves the executive secretary function for the Agency's Medications Development Workgroup.

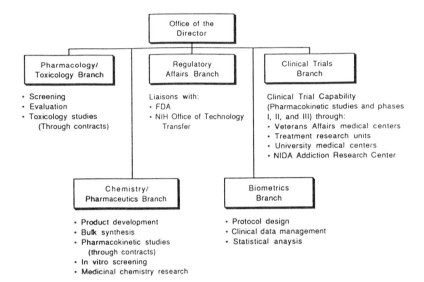

FIGURE B.1 Organizational structure of MDD. SOURCE: Federal Register 57(220): 53907. November 13, 1992.

Appendix C

Diagnostic Criteria for Psychoactive Substance Dependence

TABLE C.1 Diagnostic Criteria for Psychoactive Substance Dependence (DSM-III-R)

A. At least three of the following:

1. substance often taken in larger amounts or over a longer period than the person intended
2. persistent desire or one or more unsuccessful efforts to cut down or control substance use
3. a great deal of time spent in activities necessary to get the substance (e.g., theft), taking the substance (e.g., chain smoking), or recovering from its effects
4. frequent intoxication or withdrawal symptoms when expected to fulfill major role obligations at work, school, or home (e.g., does not go to work because hung over, goes to school or work "high", intoxicated while taking care of his or her children), or when substance use is physically hazardous (e.g., drives when intoxicated)
5. important social, occupational, or recreational activities given up or reduced because of substance use
6. continued substance use despite knowledge of having a persistent or recurrent social, physiological, or physical problem that is caused or exacerbated by the use of the substance (e.g., keeps heroin despite family arguments about it, cocaine-induced depression, or having an ulcer made worse by drinking)

(continued)

211

TABLE C.1 *(continued)*

7. marked tolerance: need for markedly increased amounts of the substance (i.e., at least a 50 percent increase) in order to achieve intoxication or desired effect, or markedly diminished effect with continued use of the same amount

Note: The following items may not apply to cannabis, hallucinogens, or phencyclidine (PCP):

8. characteristic withdrawal symptoms (see specific withdrawal syndromes under Psychoactive Substance-induced Organic Mental Disorders)
9. substance often taken to relieve or avoid withdrawal symptoms

B. Some symptoms of the disturbance have persisted for at least 1 month, or have occurred repeatedly over a longer period of time.

Criteria for severity of psychoactive substance dependence

Mild: Few, if any, symptoms in excess of those required to make the diagnosis, and the symptoms result in no more than mild impairment in occupational functioning or in usual social activities or relationships with others.

Moderate: Symptoms or functional impairment between "mild" and "severe"

Severe: Many symptoms in excess of those required to make the diagnosis, and the symptoms markedly interfere with occupational functioning or with usual social activities or relationships with others.[a]

In Partial Remission: During the past six months, some use of the substance and some symptoms of dependence

In Full Remission: During the past six months, either no use of the substance, or use of the substance and no symptoms of dependence.

[a]Because of the availability of cigarettes and other nicotine-containing substances and the absence of a clinically significant nicotine intoxication syndrome, impairment in occupational or social functioning is not necessary for a rating of severe Nicotine Dependence.

SOURCE: American Psychiatric Association. 1987. Diagnostic and Statistical Manual of Mental Disorders, 3rd ed. revised (DSM-III-R). Washington, DC: American Psychiatric Association.

TABLE C.2   Diagnostic Criteria for Psychoactive Substance Abuse (ICD-10 Draft)

Flx. 2 Dependence syndrome

A cluster of physiological, behavioral and cognitive phenomena in which the use of a substance or a class of substances takes on a much higher priority for a given individual than the other behaviors that once had higher value. A central descriptive characteristic of the dependence syndrome is the desire (often strong, sometimes overpowering) to take drugs (which may or may not have been medically prescribed), alcohol or tobacco. There may be evidence that return to substance use after a period of abstinence leads to a more rapid reappearance of other features of the syndrome than occurs with non-dependent individuals.

Diagnostic guidelines

A definite diagnosis of dependence should usually only be made if three or more of the following have been experienced or exhibited at some time during the previous year:

    (i)   A strong desire or sense of compulsion to take the substance.

    (ii)   An impaired capacity to control substance-taking behavior in terms of its onset, termination, or levels of use.

    (iii)   Substance use with the intention of relieving withdrawal symptoms and with awareness that this strategy is effective.

    (iv)   A physiological withdrawal state (see .4 and .5)

    (v)   Evidence of tolerance such that increased doses of the substance are required in order to achieve effects originally produced by lower doses. (Clear examples of this are found in alcohol and opiate dependent individuals who may take daily doses of the substance sufficient to incapacitate or kill non-tolerant users.)

    (vi)   A narrowing of the personal repertoire of patterns of substance use (e.g., a tendency to drink alcoholic drinks in the same way on weekdays and weekends and whatever the social constraints regarding appropriate drinking behavior).

    (vii)   Progressive neglect of alternative pleasures or interests in favor of substance use.

    (viii)   Persisting with substance use despite clear evidence of overtly harmful consequences. (Adverse consequences may be medical as with harm to the liver through excessive drinking, social as in the case of loss of a job through drug-related impairment of performance, or psychological as in the case of depressive mood states consequent to periods of heavy substance use).

(continued)

TABLE C.2 *(continued)*

It is an essential characteristic of the dependence syndrome that either substance taking or a desire to take a particular substance should be present; the subjective awareness of compulsion to use drugs is most commonly seen during attempts to stop or control substance use. This diagnostic requirement would exclude, for instance, surgical patients given opiate drugs for the relief of pain and who may show signs of an opiate withdrawal state when drugs are not given, but who have no desire to continue taking drugs.

The dependence syndrome may be present for a specific substance (e.g., tobacco or diazepam), for a class of substances (e.g., opiate and opioid drugs); or for a wider range of different substances (as for those individuals who feel a sense of compulsion regularly to use whatever drugs are available and who show distress, agitation, and/or physical signs of a withdrawal stat upon abstinence).

Includes: chronic alcoholism; dipsomania; drug addiction NOS.

The diagnosis of the dependence syndrome may be further specified by the following fifth character codes:

Flx.20	Currently abstinent
Flx.21	Currently abstinent, but in a protected environment (e.g., in hospital, in a therapeutic community, in prison, etc.)
Flx.22	Currently on a clinically supervised maintenance or replacement regime (e.g., with methadone; nicotine-gum or patch)
Flx.23	Currently abstinent, but receiving aversive treatment on aversive blocking drugs (e.g. naltrexone or disulfiram)
Flx.24	Currently using the substance
Flx.25	Continuous use
Flx.26	Episodic use (dipsomania)

SOURCE: World Health Organization. 1990. Draft of chapter V: mental and behavioural disorders. Clinical descriptions and diagnostic guidelines. International Classification of Diseases, 10th rev. Geneva: WHO. As cited in: O'Brien CP, Jaffe JH, eds. Addictive States. New York: Raven Press.

Appendix D

Survey of Pharmaceutical Companies

To aid the committee in assessing the incentives and disincentives to the pharmaceutical industry's investment in research and development in the field of anti-addiction medications, a questionnaire was sent by the Pharmaceutical Manufacturers Association, the Generic Pharmaceutical Industry Association, and the Biotechnology Industry Organization to their members currently involved with central nervous system medications. The questionnaire was developed by the committee and IOM staff in conjunction with the industry organizations. Responses were blinded and the committee did not have information on the company or the job title of the survey respondent. A total of 19 responses were received, and the responses were viewed by the committee as indicative but not definitive.

Figure D.1 indicates how respondents rated the uncertainty or risk involved in R&D issues in the field of drug addiction as compared with the fields of cancer, AIDS, and cardiovascular disease. Clearly, these results are not a quantitative assessment of the industry, but the drug-addiction field is perceived to be high risk in all areas except for likelihood of competitive advantage over other treatments and likelihood of fast track FDA review. The committee used the survey solely as a point of reference and a starting point for committee and individual discussions with representatives of the pharmaceutical industry.

Questionnaire on Factors Influencing Pharmaceutical Companies' Investment in R&D in Medications for Treating Illicit Drug Abuse

The names of individual respondents or their firms will not be given to the IOM Committee or be included in the Committee's report.

(Responses are tabulated or are in bold type)

1. Has your company <u>ever had</u> a <u>drug discovery program</u> in any of the following areas?

a. cocaine/crack addiction	Yes 3	No 16
b. heroin dependence	Yes 4	No 15
c. alcoholism	Yes 5	No 13
d. nicotine addiction	Yes 3	No 14

2. Has your company <u>ever had</u> a <u>drug development or in-licensing effort</u> in any of the following areas?

a. cocaine/crack addiction	Yes 3	No 14
b. heroin dependence	Yes 3	No 13
c. alcoholism	Yes 6	No 11
d. nicotine addiction	Yes 6	No 11

3. If your company has <u>never had</u> a drug discovery or drug development/in-licensing program in one or more of these areas, please indicate the area and the major reason(s) for this decision.

a. role of the potential market 6
b. federal regulations 2
c. state, local or community barriers 1
d. difficulty in conducting clinical trials 4
e. other reasons (please state/explain)

- **Beyond current focus on neurological disorders**
- **Drug discovery (and development) is not defined in the current mission of our business**
- **Other project opportunities/priorities and resources**
- **Not in area of expertise/experience**
- **Lack of preclinical leads**

- Concern that use of a drug for "abuse" treatment might tarnish its image for other uses
  - Outside our area of expertise
  - Indication(s) lay outside our areas of strategic interest.

4(a). If your company once had a drug discovery or drug development/in-licensing program in one or more of these areas but no longer does, please indicate the area and state the major reason(s) for dropping the program.

- Alcoholism program dropped due to market potential
- High recidivism
- Community concept that drugs shouldn't be used to cure an addiction
- Nicotine addiction-loss of commercial interest due to unfavorable marketing experience with other products (nicotine transdermal patches)
- No further leads at this time, would review alcohol or nicotine programs for any leads.

(b). What incentives (including legislative proposals) would be necessary for your company to renew its effort in those areas (please state area)?

- R&D tax credits
- Guaranteed market exclusivity for ten years or more
- Availability of government sponsored patents on an exclusive basis
- Guaranteed pricing freedom to achieve high margins to enable re-investment in R&D, educational programs, and broad marketing
- None, no commercial interest
- Sponsor preclinical support
- Reclassification of many schedule I drugs to schedule II
- Indemnification for usage in subject populations

5. If your company has a drug discovery or drug development/in-licensing program for medications to treat drug abuse please state the positive incentives that attracted you to this field. (NOTE: We are referring primarily to medications to treat cocaine and opiate addictions).

- Drug being evaluated has potential for analgesia. This is our primary commercial interest

- Urgency of medical need—rapid approvability and demand for effective therapy
- Our drug discovery program, re: cocaine abuse, involves interaction with MDD-NIDA, and NIH to search our existing compound file for potentially useful compounds. Incentive was statement by Senator Biden to Mr. George Sella (then PMA chairman). Our only current incentive is scientific interest, and good relations.
- We decided to invest $10M or so in alcohol and nicotine due to good lead and its public health importance-program does work for both.
- Large patient population, public good.
- Large unmet medical need.
- Significant experience in treating nicotine addiction shows that programs can be commercially viable.

6. Are you aware of NIDA's Medications Development Division (MDD)?

　　　yes 14　　　　no 5

7. Are you aware of NIDA's preclinical screening program?

　　　yes 12　　　　no 4　　　　vaguely 1

8. What is your perspective on the role of NIDA's MDD?

- MDD has expressed considerable interest, is in position to provide considerable support for our project.
- No major accomplishments to date
- Could be very useful.
- It is viewed as a major deterrent to discovery/development efforts by companies like ours, because of 1) likelihood of government involvement in pricing, 2) concerns re: government being involved in the "go/no go" development decision-making and 3) involvement of taxpayer dollars.
- Excellent approach to this problem. Highly productive.
- To evaluate potential drugs, particularly those well along in development, for use in the treatment of cocaine addiction (antagonists to cocaine, or drugs as adjuncts to psychotherapy).
- NIDA's investment is helpful to industry to explore uses of drugs already in development as well as assist in exploration of early leads from related research programs in industry.
- Very useful, underutilized.

- Generally involve CRADAs with "fair pricing" provisions and thus not usable.
- Already working with NIDA in a constructive collaboration.
- Waste of time. They are not effective. PMA companies could do a better job if there were an incentive.

9. Please add any additional comments that you feel would assist the Institute of Medicine's Committee on Medications Development and Research at the National Institute on Drug Abuse to better understand the incentives and disincentives for private sector R&D involvement in producing medications to treat illicit drug abuse (particularly cocaine and opiate addictions).

- Development of medications to treat drug abuse is perceived to be of low commercial value. Therefore, direct financial support or co-development is essential to provide sufficient incentive.
- Speaking as a member of a firm not involved in any programs, but strictly as an outside observer, disincentives are enormous when the proposed new compound becomes entrapped in DEA's scheduling system. These barriers should be changed.
- Increase transparency.
- Offer consultative support to ongoing industrial research efforts.
- We have concerns about handing over control of the product development decision making to NIDA along with the official involvement of pricing, plus the likelihood of "unofficial" pressures to continue development even if the sponsor wished to discontinue. The involvement of tax dollars in "for-profit" drug development projects by pharmaceutical companies is also viewed as risky in today's political climate.
- Adequate patent protection is essential.
- Avoidance of accusations of collusion with a government agency.
- Recognition of altruism in cooperative ventures.
- Have FDA run DEA.
- Change many Schedule I drugs to Schedule II.
- Eliminate "fair pricing" clause from HHS CRADAs.
- The primary disincentive is that your medication (the company's) is the only one with a traceable history. The subjects treated not only may have concomitant ethical pharmaceuticals, but also drugs of questionable origin and purity. Drug/drug interactions, unexpected adverse interactions due to prior history of usage leave only the company vulnerable to litigation.

10. Please fill out Attachments 1 and 2.

Attachment 1

The intent of this exercise is to gain information on how pharmaceutical companies view the drug abuse area in relation to other project areas, with respect to certain factors commonly used to judge R&D priorities. (**NOTE**: By "drug abuse area" we mean illicit drug use, primarily in the form of opiate and cocaine addictions, we do not mean use of alcohol, nicotine, or abuse of prescription drugs.)

Please put a number from 1 to 5 in each blank, based on the scale below.

1-------------------2-------------------3-------------------4-------------------5
High uncertainty   Average uncertainty   Low uncertainty
or risk   or risk   or risk

Cancer _____   Drug Abuse _____   AIDS _____   Cardiovascular _____

These four disease categories were repeated in the survey for each of the following 12 areas. The responses are displayed in Figure D.1.

1. Sufficient scientific knowledge of disease to begin a drug discovery/drug development program

2. Availability of screening techniques and animal models

3. Clear efficacy endpoints for ethical studies

4. Availability of qualified clinical investigators

5. Likelihood of fast track review or special handling by FDA

6. Patentability of product

7. Product liability risk

8. Sufficient market size

9. Likelihood of competitive advantage over other treatments

10. Adequate price and reliable reimbursement

11. Sufficient projected return on investment

12. Good public image; intangible benefits to company or other company products.

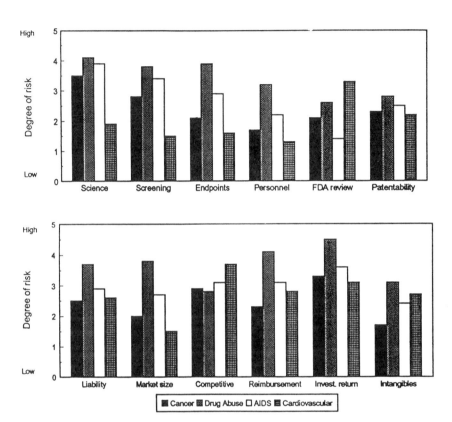

Figure D.1 Survey results. Issues involved in R&D were ranked for four diseases: cancer, drug addiction, AIDS, and cardiovascular disease (see Attachment 1 of the survey).

Attachment 2
POLICY SUGGESTIONS

For each box in Attachment 1 in which you put a 1 or 2 for Drug Abuse, i.e., for each factor for which you think the Drug Abuse area is handicapped by higher-than-average uncertainty or risk, please state briefly what you would recommend to improve the situation. Suggestions should be one-liners (e.g., "amend the Orphan Drug Act to include all drugs intended for drug abuse", "increase the basic science budget at NIDA by $50 million per year," "change regulations requiring . . .", etc.).

The intent is not to get fully evaluated policy recommendations that are formally approved by your company but rather to get your personal ideas for further consideration. Please treat this as a "brainstorming by mail" or a "public policy suggestion box". No individual attributions will be given to the IOM Committee on Medications Development and Research at NIDA.

1. Basic scientific knowledge
   • **More emphasis on underlying biochemical mechanisms needed.**
   • **Not a high profile research area, nor widely viewed as attractive.**
   • **Improve quality and focus of ongoing research, especially in molecular biology of addictive process.**
   • **What is molecular basis of addiction.**
   • **Why will addicts relapse on drug therapy.**
   • **Fund special NIDA extramural research efforts via executive branch edict or legislation.**
   • **Need further mechanistic work, availability of modern day screens, etc.**
   • **Inter-company interaction should be encouraged.**
   • **Increase NIDA budget.**
   • **Increase NIH support of this domain of research.**
   • **Increase NIDA budget.**
   • **Fund biotech startups.**

2. Screening techniques and animal models
   • **Technically demanding and applicability to humans not certain.**
   • **Do not over-rely on these; expedite pathway to clinic with good hypotheses.**
   • **Good models are lacking.**
   • **Fund special NIDA extramural research efforts.**
   • **Increase NIDA budget.**

- More money to MDD-NIDA, the process is now painfully slow.
- Primates too expensive-develop in vitro screens?
- Start search for susceptibility genes.
- Develop transgenic animals with increased "abuse liability."

3. Efficacy endpoints

- Since there are both psychological as well as physiological dependencies at work, a clear endpoint especially on the psychological aspects would be difficult.
- Clear FDA guidelines would help.
- Do not ask drug to do everything—acute drug effects in many cases will be combined with long term counselling to keep patient clean.
- Develop NIDA/FDA/industry consensus guidelines for study requirements and officially-recognized endpoints.
- Movement to clinical trials should be accelerated.
- Very difficult to improve.
- No clear standards except very expensive followup surrogates.
- Need more validation of surrogate endpoints.

4. Availability of qualified clinical investigators

- The field is not one to attract the best medical school faculty.
- A general problem in psychotherapeutics—particularly acute drug dependence. Need more physicians; scientists.
- Consider an investigative network similar to the ACTG mechanism for anti-HIV treatments.
- Training and research support need improvement.

5. FDA review

- Not certain of FDA's view of this area.
- An FDA fast track is based on disease slate vs. availability of existing treatments. This in my opinion, would not warrant FDA's highest attention (over drugs in categories of AIDS or cancer treatment).
- Expedite.
- Declare substance-abuse drugs and biologicals "AA" priority, like AIDS drugs.
- Safety should be the major criterion, with efficacy being a clinical finding; e.g. more flexibility in evaluating animal pharmacology should be allowed.
- Automatic priority ranking for any drug with significant lower abuse of target agents.

- Safety a real problem in the treated population. FDA will be all over drug interactions and serious adverse reactions.

6. Patent protection
- No special issues—use patents for psychotherapeutics discovered for other indications will be common.
- Give (via legislation) substance-abuse drugs Waxman-Hatch type exclusivity/patent life extension.
- The patent office must recognize the speculative nature of current research when evaluating relevance of animal testing data.

7. Product liability
- Side effects of CNS drugs used long term.
- High-unstable patient population leads to high potential for adverse events (which can easily be non-drug related).
- Government indemnification, as for vaccines, should be provided.
- Insurance pool—similar to vaccines—for products intended to treat drug liability.
- Government should subsidize insurance costs for adverse drug effects during testing and clinical use.
- Government assumption of risk.
- Tort reform.
- Use legislation to eliminate lawyers.
- Who do you sue—the company or the guy on the end of the block with the gun?

8. Market size
- Hard to identify or characterize.
- Potentially large, but returns on investments may be poor if reimbursement not forthcoming in managed care—most patients are financially distressed.
- Supportive therapy is used to exclusion of drug therapy.
- Candidates can't afford intensive medical therapy.
- May not be a problem if government reimburses. Tied up in health care reform, pricing, etc.
- Patient unreliability is the big problem, possibly address by creating a national network between drug treatment centers and programs.
- Out-licensing partners should be sought; smaller returns become more meaningful (profitable) to smaller, lower overhead operations.

- If primary purchaser is government, insures no tax or rebate, free market pricing.
- Increase percent of "war on drugs" billions that goes to treatment. Spend less on enforcement—reduce the demand for illicit drugs by effective treatment programs.

9. Competitive advantage
- No effective therapies available for any addiction.
- Reduce the disincentive and sponsors may be willing to seek products with advantages.
- Company that loses out because of competition by a selected drug should receive some compensation.
- Free market.
- Try more experimental approaches.

10. Price and reimbursement
- Not sure who is going to pay.
- Ensure pricing that would allow sufficient return on investment.
- Typically, it would be my opinion that these patients may not be under routine care of a PCP or have their own insurance/ability to pay.
- Expect unreasonable political pressure to have low prices because of government subsidy to research or reimbursement.
- Very uncertain, due to Health Care Reform, but protection from direct and indirect price caps, e.g., by legislation exemption, substance-abuse treatments, is essential.
- Government support for high prices.
- Tax advantages would have to support the low prices necessitated by this class of drug.
- Make drug treatment programs mandatory part of HMO and insurance industry payment programs.
- Federal and state government—primary customer.

11. Return on investment
- Not well understood.
- May be difficult to determine length of time of recovery for ROI.
- Government interference and negative image of drug therapy will not provide reasonable margins.
- Will this be completely reimbursed?
- Costs of development should be distributed among "partners" e.g. government, venture capital.

12. Public image and intangibles
- Publish NIDA's work at a more high profile level.
- A mixed area: charging the typical drug abuser for therapy will be seen negatively.
- "Substitute addictions" will be invented by the press for successful therapies.
- Remove the disincentives, so that the prospects of bad publicity, poor pricing, etc. no longer outweigh the goodwill that would accrue for sponsors of successful treatments or preventive measures.
- Could work around this problem if had clear benefits.
- Get the current administration to spend less time bashing the pharmaceutical industry.
- Too visible an arena, much like AIDS. Too susceptible to government/Congress trying to make "political" points on pricing at the same time crying about lack of treatment. It's a no win situation.

Other comments:
- Drug efficacy must be assessed in the context of overall care for the addict; clinical studies isolating drug from other modalities may set unrealistically high hurdles.
- I think the major problem is no science in this area.
- The PMA seems to be focusing on the business aspect of this project, while interactions are mainly at the scientific level. What is absolutely essential at this time is a forum to share compounds and data, and to worry about "who will develop?" later. NIH-Addiction Research Center should also be involved with companies; that funnel compounds to MDD-NIDA at this time. An excellent forum is the College on Problems of Drug Dependence (CPDD). Their involvement in any such venture is extremely helpful.
- Trials a special problem of compliance and longterm followup. Although NIH could help fund, their behavior on CRADAs makes this unattractive re #10 and #11 above.
- Make NIDA/industry collaborations better and really allow industry to make a reasonable return on investment.

Appendix E

Model Federal Programs in Pharmaceutical R&D

The federal government sponsors 13 pharmaceutical research and development programs (OTA, 1993). The programs cover a wide array of fields, including drug addiction, cancer, malaria, and contraception. This appendix describes several selected programs that have successfully brought medications to market with the cooperation of commercial sponsors: the Antiepileptic Drug Development Program of the National Institute of Neurological Disorders and Stroke (NINDS) and the cancer-drug and AIDS-drug discovery and development programs of the National Cancer Institute (NCI) and the National Institute of Allergy and Infectious Diseases (NIAID) (Table E.1). Most of the information obtained in this appendix was based on interviews with leaders of the programs (see Appendix A). The goal of identifying the successful elements of the programs is to help the Medications Development Division (MDD) of the National Institute on Drug Abuse shape the future of its program.

ANTIEPILEPTIC DRUG DEVELOPMENT PROGRAM

Background

The Antiepileptic Drug Development Program (ADD) was created in 1975 to encourage the development of medications to treat epilepsy, which afflicts 2 million Americans. As early as 1968, when Congress asked the federal government to make more drugs available, the National Institutes of Health

(NIH) responded by launching an initiative that eventually resulted in the formation of the ADD. The program is now situated within the Epilepsy Branch of NINDS. Its current budget of about $4 million is spent on extramural contracts administered by a staff of 21. The market for anti-epilepsy drugs is estimated at $300—500 million.

When the program was created, drugs were available to treat epilepsy; but despite optimal dosing, about 10 percent of patients still experienced seizures. In addition, many patients suffered from side effects. There was no apparent industry interest in developing more-effective and less-toxic medications. The program was designed to stimulate the private sector by providing incentives to develop and market a new generation of antiepilepsy drugs. The incentives offered by the ADD were to share funding and to offer expertise, such as in the design, monitoring, or analysis of a clinical trial (Kupferberg, 1990).

In the early years of the ADD, its resources were devoted almost entirely to controlled clinical trials. The program pioneered new outcome measures designed to evaluate a drug's efficacy in a clinical trial. These novel approaches to establishing efficacy required fewer patients to be studied over a shorter period and so were less expensive. Two drugs that were on the market in Europe, carbamazepine and valproic acid, were the first tested by the ADD in clinical trials and were found effective. By the middle 1970s, the clinical data contributed to the acquisition of Food and Drug Administration (FDA) marketing approval for the ADD's industry partners.

The program began a preclinical screening component in 1974. Industry provided the ADD with most of the chemicals, which are screened at no charge and for which companies retain patent rights. Since the creation of the preclinical screening program, 17,000 chemicals have been tested. Two of them have reached or are about to reach the marketplace. The time between discovery and marketing approval for those two successful chemicals was about 12 years.

The program's resources are divided almost equally between preclinical research and clinical trials. The preclinical research primarily supports preclinical screening and toxicity testing to determine target-organ toxicity. The clinical trials are sponsored by contract at academic medical centers. Because of innovations in clinical trial design, each trial normally requires fewer than 200 patients. The smaller trials (usually Phase I and II trials) are used to establish safety and to gain enough efficacy information to attract an industry partner that can sponsor larger trials. The larger trials, which build on the smaller ones, are necessary for FDA regulatory requirements.

TABLE E.1 Model Federal Pharmaceutical Research and Development Programs

Program	Type of Research	Year Begun	FY93 Budget ($ millions)	FTEs[a]
Epilepsy[b]		1975		
Antiepileptic Drug Development Program	Preclinical and clinical extramural		4	21
Cancer[c]		1955		
Developmental Therapeutics Program	Preclinical extramural and intramural		58	212
Cancer Therapy Evaluation Program	Clinical extramural		181	55
Clinical Oncology Program	Clinical intramural		52	360
AIDS[d]		1987		
Basic Research and Development Program	Preclinical extramural		60	90[e]
Clinical Research Program	Clinical extramural and intramural		125[f]	
Treatment Research Operations Program	Clinical extramural and intramural			

[a]Number of full-time equivalent personnel.
[b]Epilepsy Branch, NINDS.
[c]Division of Cancer Treatment, NCI.
[d]Division of AIDS, NIAID.
[e] Number of full-time equivalents for all three AIDS drug discovery and development programs.
[f] Combined budget for Clinical Research and Treatment Research Operations Program.

Elements of Success

Over the course of almost 20 years, the program has succeeded, in conjunction with drug companies, in bringing at least six drugs to market. The varied medications now available to treat epilepsy are so effective for patients that drug companies, perceiving the market to be saturated, have become less interested in working with the ADD. Not resting on its laurels, the ADD is now in the process of changing its direction to an entirely new and unexplored arena: medications to prevent epilepsy symptoms.

Program administrators have attributed their success to the following factors:

• *The existence of animal models.* Animal models for epilepsy have been indispensable in all fields of research, such as for screening tests to search for potential treatments and for assessing drug efficacy, mechanism of action, toxicity, and side effects.

• *Strong support from constituency groups.* The Epilepsy Foundation of America, whose membership exceeds 20,000, has been very supportive of the ADD. It has been instrumental in ensuring stable financial support from Congress.

• *Strong support from industry.* Industry has provided the ADD with about 1,000 chemicals per year for preclinical screening. It has also been interested in working with the ADD in clinical trials and in seeking guidance on drug development.

•   *Realistic expectations.* The program's leadership has worked constructively with Congress to ensure that the ADD's goals remain realistic in light of its resources. The pressure to produce results on an unreasonable schedule is less than that in the case of medications for drug addiction because the social burdens created by epilepsy are not as severe as those created by drug addiction.

• *Large market size.* The market for an antiepilepsy drug is estimated at $300-500 million, which is sufficient to attract pharmaceutical companies to work with the ADD. The reimbursement climate has also been advantageous.

• *Favorable regulatory climate.* FDA has been receptive to the need to increase availability of antiepilepsy medications. The ADD enjoys good working relationships with FDA staff.

• *Medically defined outcome measures.* Clinical trials are aided by readily identifiable, medically acceptable outcome measures of drug efficacy. This has led to new clinical-trial designs that can establish efficacy with fewer patients at lower cost.

NATIONAL CANCER INSTITUTE CANCER-DRUG
DISCOVERY AND DEVELOPMENT PROGRAMS

Background

NCI sponsors the largest and oldest drug discovery and development program in the federal government. The NCI program was established in 1955 as the Cancer Chemotherapy National Service Center to fill a need that was not being addressed by either universities or industry. As the program grew, it was divided into several programs in NCI's Division of Cancer Treatment, where they are now. The programs in the division support an increasingly broad spectrum of preclinical and clinical research. In collaboration with industry, the programs strive to make new cancer treatments available. The preclinical screening programs have evaluated over 450,000 chemicals in almost 40 years of testing. NCI's systematic commitment to all aspects of drug development has resulted in the approval of 48 drugs—the majority of commercially available cancer treatments—including methotrexate, doxorubicin, and vincristine (Zubrod et al., 1977; Grever et al., 1992).

Today's commercial market for anticancer drugs depends on the incidence of the cancer in question and many other factors. The market for a given drug is estimated at anywhere from $1 million to $500 million. NCI's investment will depend on a drug's therapeutic promise, the size of the potential market, and the resources of its commercial partner.

All 5 programs in the NCI Division of Cancer Treatment play a role, but three of them are most germane to drug discovery and development. Most of the preclinical research is in the Developmental Therapeutics Program, which had a FY 1993 budget of about $58 million and staff of 212. Most of the clinical research is supported under the Cancer Therapy Evaluation Program and the Clinical Oncology Program, which had a combined FY 1993 budget of about $233 million. These three programs are described below.

Preclinical Research

The Developmental Therapeutics Program performs a broad spectrum of preclinical research to identify promising cancer medications. This research is undertaken by nine extramural branches and five intramural laboratories. Its contract screening program alone evaluates the potential therapeutic value of about 10,000 new chemicals each year. A revised screening battery, modified in 1985, subjects each chemical to tests against 60 human-tumor cell lines derived from seven cancer types (lung, colon, melanoma, renal, ovarian, brain, and leukemia). After reviewing the results from these in vitro tests, a special committee determines what secondary in vitro and in vivo studies are warranted. About 4 percent of chemicals screened by the program have been referred for further testing (Grever et al., 1992). The program also screens antiviral drugs that may show promise in combating HIV infection and AIDS.

The screening program acquires chemicals from industry and academe in almost equal proportions. The testing is performed at no cost to the sponsor. In the standard screening agreement, NCI stipulates that its testing does not constitute "invention" under the patent laws and thereby cedes intellectual property rights to the sponsor. Results are kept confidential unless the chemical is pursued in clinical trials. When the decision is made to proceed to clinical trials, the sponsor is given 1 year to file a patent before the screening results are released (M. Grever, NCI, personal communication).

Among the many unique screening program resources supported by NCI is the Natural Product Repository. In recognition that natural products have contributed to many of the currently used anticancer agents, this repository contains almost 70,000 extracts of natural products systematically collected worldwide by NCI contractors. Taxol, one of NCI's most recent and important contributions to cancer treatment, was collected under this program in the early 1960s.

In addition to the screening program, the Developmental Therapeutics Program supports many other preclinical tasks. In its preclinical pharmacology research, it develops analytic methods to determine drug concentrations and metabolites in animals. This provides critical data about drug and metabolite excretion or clearance for use in later human testing. In its formulation research, it strives to ensure that potential medications have bioavailability in humans, especially at the target site. In some cases, this requires the modification of an otherwise insoluble agent to an active species. Finally, in its preclinical toxicology research, it examines acute and subacute toxicity of test chemicals in various animal species.

Clinical Research

Clinical research is supported in two complementary programs: the Cancer Therapy Evaluation Program, which supports extramural research, and the Clinical Oncology Program, which supports intramural research. Together, these programs were budgeted in FY 1993 at about $233 million.

The Cancer Therapy Evaluation Program supports a large national network of clinical oncology cooperative groups at hospitals and other clinical sites. The FY 1993 budget was about $179 million. The groups provide state-of-the-art care for patients and participate in clinical trials designed to develop better cancer therapies. The program consists of more than 300 hospitals and community clinics and nearly 2500 physicians. In FY 1993, about 800 protocols were used to investigate the therapeutic potential of some 200 new therapies alone or in combination with approved drugs. Of those 800 protocols, 150 involved Phase III clinical trials. The cooperative agreements that fund the cooperative groups support data management, investigational-drug costs (if any), and quality assurance, but they do not provide funds for patient care. Almost 75 percent of the new drugs being studied by the groups are provided by industry, 10 percent are provided by university researchers, and about 10 percent come from the Division of Cancer Treatment's preclinical research sponsored by the Developmental Therapeutics Program. Statistical and regulatory support to aid research design and approvals is in the program's Biometrics Research Branch and Regulatory Affairs Branch, respectively.

The Clinical Oncology Program, funded in FY 1993 at $53 million, is based at NIH's Clinical Center. Not only does this program conduct clinical trials of cancer treatments, but it also conducts trials of treatments for cancers associated with AIDS, such as Kaposi's sarcoma.

Elements of Success

Since the creation of the program, the NCI has contributed to the marketing of 48 anticancer drugs. That figure constitutes more than half of all U.S. drugs marketed to treat cancer.

Program administrators have attributed their success to the following factors:

- *Clinical-trials capacity.* Through the clinical oncology cooperative groups and the NIH Clinical Center, NCI supports a vast network of over 300 hospitals and 2,500 physicians. Thousands of new patients each year can take advantage of NCI-supported clinical trials.
- *Adequate resources.* In almost 40 years of existence, NCI's drug discovery and development programs have received sufficient resources (funding and personnel) to develop a large infrastructure. The programs have the capacity to perform every phase of drug development, from test tube to clinic, except bulk manufacturing, marketing, and distribution.
- *Animal models.* Many cancer treatments have been identified with the aid of animal models for particular tumor types. An animal model can be used in preclinical screening and in assessing drug efficacy, toxicity, mechanism of action and side effects.
- *Advances in basic research.* For years, NCI has had a strong commitment to understanding the molecular biology of malignant

transformation. This basic-research investment is expected to yield numerous innovations in drug development.

   •   *Confidentiality of screening results.* Industry provides NCI with an average of 5,000 chemicals per year for screening. NCI's standard screening agreement used to acquire chemicals assures the sponsor complete confidentiality except when a chemical shows clinical promise, in which case the sponsor is given 1 year to file a patent application before the results are made public.

   •   *Favorable regulatory climate.* NCI has experienced long-standing collegial relations with FDA. In addition, many anticancer drugs have benefited from special expedited review by FDA because they qualify under recent FDA regulations as treatments for serious or life-threatening diseases.

   •   *Support of constituency groups.* Constituency groups have for years worked with Congress and the executive branch to play a vigorous role in support of NCI research. NCI enjoys the largest budget of all NIH institutes and submits its annual budget directly to the President in what is called a bypass budget to avoid competition with other health programs.

   •   *Staff commitment.* The Division of Cancer Treatment has benefited from a vigilant commitment of its staff to bring drugs for cancer treatment to market.

NATIONAL INSTITUTE OF ALLERGY AND INFECTIOUS DISEASES DRUG DISCOVERY AND DEVELOPMENT PROGRAMS

Background

Antiviral and anti-infection drugs to treat AIDS are the focus of research and development programs of the NIAID. Created in 1987, these programs were designed to work with university and private researchers to bring drugs quickly to market to treat both HIV infection and the opportunistic infections afflicting AIDS patients.

The commercial market for antiviral and anti-infection drugs for HIV and AIDS-related disease depends on the indication. There has been robust commercial response, to judge the fact that 74 companies now have 103 medications in clinical trials or awaiting regulatory approval at FDA (PMA, 1993). The 1992 domestic sales of AZT (zidovudine) resulted in $195 million in revenues to the manufacturer (P. Arno, Albert Einstein College of Medicine, personal communication). NIAID's Division of AIDS sponsors three programs that are collectively committed to the discovery and development of AIDS drugs. The budget for the three programs in FY 1993 totaled about $185 million, $60 million for preclinical research and $125 million for clinical research. About 90 full-time equivalent staff administer this total budget.

Preclinical Research

The division's Basic Research and Development Program is responsible for preclinical research on AIDS antiviral and anti-infection treatments. Through extramural grants, contracts, and cooperative agreements, this program has an innovative goal: to facilitate the development of drugs, immunity modulators, gene therapies, and other novel treatments through the support of high-risk basic and applied research that is unlikely to be supported by the private sector. Basic research is not usually supported in most other federal research and development programs, but the novelty of this program is that it links basic research with drug development and clinical research. The program does not support screening tests, because all preclinical screening of AIDS antiviral drugs is performed separately by NCI.

The cooperative agreements supported by the Basic Research and Development Program are the vehicles used to bring university and industry researchers together to work on multidisciplinary preclinical research, both basic and applied. The cooperative agreements fund national cooperative drug discovery groups (NCDDGs) that strive to identify treatments for HIV infection and the opportunistic infections associated with AIDS. The cooperative agreements constitute about 20 percent of the program's $60 million budget.

The Basic Research and Development Program, though relatively young, already has witnessed some success: it has sponsored the preclinical research leading to clinical trials for six new medications. One of these innovative medications is a non-nucleoside inhibitor of HIV reverse transcriptase, bisheteroarylpiperazine (BHAP), which is being developed with Upjohn.

Clinical Research

All AIDS-related clinical research is supported by two programs in the Division of AIDS: the Clinical Research Program and the Treatment Research Operations Program. Together, these programs support the largest network capable of performing all types of clinical trials for AIDS therapies. Budgeted at approximately $125 million, the research is supported mostly extramurally at universities, medical centers, and community programs and intramurally at NIH's Clinical Center.

The bulk of the funds is devoted to AIDS clinical trial groups (ACTGs). ACTGs are extramural clinical-research sites that evaluate therapies for all aspects of HIV disease in adults and children, ranging from early safety studies (Phase I) to multicenter efficacy studies (Phase III). Since the creation of the network at over 50 locations, more than 23,000 patients have participated in 192 clinical studies. These studies have contributed to the approval by FDA of the three leading AIDS medications that inhibit replication of the virus: AZT, ddI (didanosine), and ddc (dideoxycytidine).

Another prominent clinical-trial network supported by the Division of AIDS is the Community Programs for Clinical Research on AIDS (CPCRA). More than 10,000 patients have been enrolled in CPCRA studies, which are conducted in such community settings as hospitals, health centers, private practices, clinics, and drug-treatment facilities. The purpose of these programs is to learn how available treatments can be used more effectively and to learn the long-term effects of treatments. For example, one CPCRA trial has found that patients intolerant to AZT can receive similar benefits from ddi and ddc. The CPCRA network is also being used to study tuberculosis treatments for people infected with both HIV and tuberculosis bacteria.

The Division also supports another kind of program, the Division of AIDS Treatment Research Initiative (DATRI). The hallmark of the DATRI is the rapid conduct of early clinical trials to propel new drugs to market.

Elements of Success

NIAID's preclinical and clinical research programs have played a pivotal role in the development of three approved AIDS antiviral drugs and most of the 49 commercially sponsored medications undergoing clinical trials for the treatment of AIDS-related opportunistic infections.

Program administrators have attributed their success to the following factors:

• *Large clinical-trial network.* The clinical research for AIDS treatments is conducted at over 200 sites nationwide. Since 1987, over 32,000 patients have participated in clinical studies. The clinical-trial network is the largest in the United States that conducts human trials of experimental AIDS therapies.

• *Linking of basic research to drug development.* A unique feature of the Division of AIDS is that it weaves together basic and applied research. The basic research is targeted to drug development through the issuance of program announcements that solicit the submission of investigator-initiated grant proposals.

• *Accepted medical treatment.* The landmark approval of AZT not only has slowed disease progression but has also proved to be an important benchmark against which to test the efficacy of promising experimental treatments.

• *Staff commitment.* NIAID staff are staunchly committed to AIDS-drug discovery and development, as evidenced by their track record of success, which is even more impressive considering that this $185 million program is administered by only 90 full-time-equivalent staff.

• *Collaboration with industry.* NIAID has experienced excellent collaborative relationships with industry. With over 1 million people infected with HIV in the United Sates and far more infected outside the United States, there has been a substantial industry interest in collaborating with NIAID in the development of antiviral and anti-infection treatments.

• *Collaboration with constituency groups.* Constituency groups have emerged as a major force in drug discovery. They have pushed NIAID to be more aggressive in the pursuit of new therapies, and they have worked with Congress to ensure that NIAID's budget expands accordingly. The relationship sometimes can be turbulent, but it is guided by mutual respect and common goals.

• *Supportive relationship with FDA.* NIAID has experienced strong support from FDA in expediting the approval of medications. FDA is invited to attend meetings between NIAID and industry informally to provide advice and technical assistance. In addition, many AIDS drugs have benefited from special expedited review by FDA because they qualify under recent FDA regulations as treatments for serious or life-threatening diseases.

• *Sponsorship of small, frequent conferences.* Innovative research ideas emerge from the division's sponsorship of eight to 12 meetings per year that bring together 70–100 researchers from universities, industry, and government.

REFERENCES

Grever MR, Schepartz SA, Chabner BA. 1992. The National Cancer Institute: cancer drug discovery and development program. Seminars in Oncology 19:622–638.

Kupferberg HJ. 1990. Preclinical drug development in the Antiepileptic Drug Development Program: a cooperative effort of government and industry. In: Meldrum BS, Williams M, eds. Current and Future Trends in Anticonvulsant, Anxiety, and Stroke Therapy. New York: Wiley-Liss. 113–130.

OTA (Office of Technology Assessment). 1993. Pharmaceutical R & D: Costs, Risks and Rewards. Washington, DC: Government Printing Office. OTA-H-522.

PMA (Pharmaceutical Manufacturers Association). 1993. AIDS Medicines: Drugs and Vaccines In Development. Washington, DC: PMA.

Zubrod CG, Schepartz SA, Carter SK. 1977. Historical background of the National Cancer Institute's drug development thrust. National Cancer Institute Monographs 45:7–11.

Appendix F

Workshop Agenda and Participants

Institute of Medicine
Committee to Study Medication Development and Research at
the National Institute on Drug Abuse

*Workshop on Policies to Stimulate Private Sector Development
of Anti-Addiction Medications*

June 13, 1994
Lecture Room, National Academy of Sciences
2101 Constitution Avenue, N.W. Washington, D.C.

WORKSHOP AGENDA

8:00–8:30 a.m. **BREAKFAST**

8:30–8:45   **OPENING REMARKS**
Laurence E. Earley, Chairman

8:45–10:45   **Panel I: Private Sector Obstacles and Opportunities**
Moderator: J. Richard Crout

Panel: Dee Gillespie, Steve Grossman,
Richard Merrill, Sherri Samotin*

10:45–12:30 **Panel II: Regulatory Issues**
Moderator: Herbert Kleber

Panel: Robert Angarola, John Coleman, George DeVaux*,
Nicholas Reuter, Frank Vocci

238

12:30–1:15   **LUNCH**

1:15–2:30   **Panel III: Research and Training Issues**
Moderator: Kathleen Foley

Panel: John Ambre, Ann Geller, Charles Grudzinskas, David Lewis*

2:30–4:00   **Panel IV: Treatment Financing Issues**
Moderator: Peter Carpenter

Panel: John Caulkins*, Jack Durell*, Eric Goplerud

4:00–5:00   **Plenary Session**

5:00   **Adjourn**

* Presenters

PARTICIPANT LIST

John Ambre
American Medical Association

Robert Angarola
Hyman, Phelps and McNamara

Gary Bennett
National Institute of
   Dental Research

Ann Carter
Drug Enforcement
   Administration

John Caulkins
RAND

John Coleman
Drug Enforcement
   Administration

Leonard Cook
National Institute on Drug Abuse

James Cooper
National Institute on Drug Abuse

Paul Coulis
National Institute on Drug Abuse

Miriam Davis
Health Policy Consultant

George DeVaux
BioDevelopment Corporation

Chris Doherty
Fox, Bennett and Turner

Jack Durell
Treatment Research Institute

Joel Egertson
National Institute on Drug Abuse

John Engel
Fox, Bennett and Turner

Susan Everingham
RAND

Lorraine Fishback
Department of Health and
   Human Services

Gretchen Freshneur
Drug Enforcement
   Administration

Jim Friedman
Substance Abuse and Mental
   Health Services Administration

Ann Geller
American Society of Addiction
   Medicine

Dee Gillespie
DuPont-Merck

Steve Grossman
Hill and Knowlton

Charles Grudzinskas
National Institute on Drug Abuse

Anthony Guarino
University of South Alabama

Thomas Heffner
Parke-Davis Pharmaceutical
  Research

James Isbister
Pharmavene, Inc.

Jerome Jaffe
Substance Abuse and Mental
  Health Services Administration

Betty Jones
Food and Drug Administration

Thomas Kuchenberg
Food and Drug Administration

Irwin Lerner
Hoffman-LaRoche

David Lewis
Brown University

Barbara McGarey
National Institutes of Health

Richard Merrill
University of Virginia
  School of Law

Jacques Normand
National Research Council

Marcy Oppenheimer
Department of Health and
  Human Services

Richard Rettig
Institute of Medicine

Nicholas Reuter
Food and Drug Administration

Barbara Roberts
Office of National Drug
  Control Policy

Sherri Samotin
Wilkerson Group, Inc.

Frank Sapienza
Drug Enforcement
  Administration

Robert Talbot-Stern
Legal Consultant

John Thomas
BioDevelopment Corporation

Frank Vocci
National Institute on Drug Abuse

Bonnie Wilford
George Washington University

Curtis Wright
Food and Drug Administration

Thomas Wyatt
National Association of
  State Controlled Substance
  Authorities

Appendix G

Health Care Reform Legislation

The 103rd Congress engaged in a landmark debate about the future scope of health care—its organization, financing, and delivery. Pharmaceutical companies participated in the national dialogue and will continue to scrutinize any future legislation. Future legislative features that are likely to have the greatest effect on private sector investment in anti-addiction medication development are:

- the degree of universal coverage (the expansion of health insurance to some or all of the uninsured);
- the inclusion of a prescription drug benefit and offsetting prescription drug rebates;
- the inclusion of drug abuse treatment benefits, and the extent to which these benefits are restricted, managed, or treated relative to other medical benefits;
- the nature of additional insurance reform, such as eliminating exclusions for preexisting conditions;
- the financing of any reforms and the measures imposed to set price controls; and
- the fate of Medicaid.

In the following paragraphs each feature is discussed to summarize its consequences for commercial development of anti-addiction medications.

UNIVERSALITY OF COVERAGE

Universal or near-universal health insurance coverage has been one goal of health care reform efforts. Only about 85 percent of the population currently has coverage under private or public health insurance (CRS, 1994). If coverage were extended to more of the uninsured, especially to those who are drug dependent, the effect would likely benefit investment in anti-addiction medications, as long as the insurance benefits are at least partially tailored to the needs of that group. Greater insurance coverage means a shift from the public funding system (primarily from block grants and state alcohol and drug agencies) to the private insurance rolls. Pharmaceutical companies prefer insurance financing rather than direct subsidies from federal and state agencies, because there is the perception that private coverage commands higher revenues. Pharmaceutical companies view insurance coverage as less risky for return on investment because private insurance coverage is more lucrative and resilient than are direct public subsidies, it increases the demand for treatment, including medication, and it increases the supply of services (thus possibly reducing waiting times for treatment) (Rogowski, 1993).

PRESCRIPTION DRUG BENEFITS

A prescription drug benefit[1] is also favorable to pharmaceutical investment in research, but not necessarily for anti-addiction medications unless future medications are non-narcotic agents. Many of the legislative proposals have included a prescription drug benefit in the minimum benefit package required of employers, and some of the proposals also extend the prescription drug benefit to the Medicare population. The inclusion of the benefit in employer health plans is forecast to have only a modest positive effect on sales because almost all employer policies already have this benefit (CBO, 1994). The expansion of the benefit to the Medicare population is far more significant because the induced demand is expected to increase pharmaceutical revenues by 4–6 percent (CBO, 1994). However, the Medicare expansion under some proposals is offset by a

---

[1]The typical prescription drug benefit offers no advantage to opiate addicts who receive daily doses of medication. The proposed benefit usually contains a $5 copayment for what is assumed to be a 30-day supply. With methadone dispensed 7 days each week and LAAM 3 days each week, due, in part, to regulatory concerns for diversion, it would be cheaper to pay for each dose out-of-pocket than to provide coverage.

proposed prescription drug rebate similar in design to the Medicaid rebate[2]. Attempting to forecast the combined effect of a Medicare expansion and rebate on pharmaceutical research and development, the Congressional Budget Office concluded that, "the returns from drug company research and development would be unlikely to change; increases resulting from one provision would wash out the decreases resulting from another" (CBO, 1994). The report also noted that a Medicare rebate might induce drug companies to shift research resources away from medications for the elderly. Pharmaceutical companies have stated their opposition to a Medicare rebate, especially because the elderly make a disproportionately high percentage of pharmaceutical purchases (PMA, 1993).

If the effect of a prescription drug benefit is to increase pharmaceutical revenues, then it should lead to more pharmaceutical research and development (R&D).[3] The large increase in pharmaceutical revenues in the 1980s was accompanied by increased investment in R&D (OTA, 1993). But there are no guarantees that additional research revenues would be devoted to developing anti-addiction medications. Throughout the 1980s, when revenues and R&D were escalating, there was such an insignificant commitment to this area that Congress enacted legislation to create a medications development research program in the National Institute on Drug Abuse (NIDA) to stimulate industry interest in anti-addiction medications (Chapter 3).

DRUG ABUSE TREATMENT BENEFITS

The scope of drug abuse benefits for treatment of addiction potentially has the greatest and most direct effect on investment in anti-addiction medications. A generous benefit would almost certainly attract more pharmaceutical investment, but because of the inability to forecast the extent of costs, benefits are generally limited to brief interventions and short-term treatment. The Health Security Act, for example, proposed coverage for up to 30 days in residential treatment or 60 days in day treatment and up to 30 outpatient psychotherapy

---

[2]Prescription drug manufacturers are required to rebate state Medicaid programs for their prescription drug purchases under the Medicaid Rebate Law, passed as part of the Omnibus Budget Reconciliation Act of 1990 (P.L. 101-508). For 1994 and thereafter, the amount of the rebate is set at 15.2 percent of the average manufacturer's price for a brand name drug and 11 percent for a generic drug.

[3]Overall, R&D expenditures have increased dramatically since 1970, although in the past year growth has slowed. In 1994, R&D is projected to increase by 9.3 percent, as compared with annual increases averaging 16 percent between 1980 and 1992 (PMA, 1993).

visits (Arons et al., 1994).[4] Such limits would not cover most of the opiate- and cocaine-dependent patients in treatment programs. Their average length of stay upon discharge is about 320 days in methadone maintenance, 47 days in residential, and 179 days in outpatient drug free programs (Batten et al., 1992). When benefits are exhausted, the patient would be shifted back to public subsidies. The current reliance on a publicly subsidized treatment system is unlikely to change (Harwood et al., 1994).

Should the benefit structure of future legislation create incentives to seek primary care instead of specialty care for treatment of drug dependence, primary care physicians will need additional training in addiction medicine. In light of the movement toward increased reliance on primary care physicians for diagnosis and treatment of all medical conditions, the committee strongly supports increased training in addiction medicine for primary care providers (Chapter 6).

INSURANCE REFORM

Management of drug abuse treatment benefits and parity of the benefit with other medical conditions hold the most favorable prospects for pharmaceutical investment. Parity of the benefit means that the coverage is not discriminatory; it is provided on the same basis as are benefits for other chronic and relapsing conditions. As described earlier, managed benefits can increase access, allowing more patients to receive appropriate treatment. The more patients that are in treatment, the greater is the demand for prescription drugs.

Drug addiction is considered a chronic, relapsing medical condition—as are asthma, hypertension, and diabetes. All of those disorders are characterized by a constellation of genetic, biological, behavioral, and environmental factors. With respect to hypertension, behavioral choices, such as ingestion of high-fat foods, failure to exercise, and non-compliance with medication, can contribute to the onset and severity of the disorder. Unfortunately, the overall similarities between drug addiction and other chronic medical disorders remain unappreciated by the general public, which sees addiction only as a failure of will power or evidence of a social disorder. The stigmatization of drug dependence and its treatment have hindered pharmaceutical development (Chapter 9).

---

[4]The Health Security Act also provided for up to 120 days of counseling in exchange for inpatient or residential coverage.

FINANCING HEALTH CARE REFORM
AND THE FATE OF MEDICAID

The financing of health care reform has been proposed to come from new taxes on tobacco, payroll taxes, and restrictions on the growth of Medicare and Medicaid spending. Medicare has such a negligible role in financing the treatment of addiction that curtailing Medicare spending is not likely to affect either the avenues of treatment or the demand for anti-addiction medications. Medicaid spending reductions carry more significance, but the outcome for development of anti-addiction medications is far from clear. Decreases in federal Medicaid spending could force the states to restrict Medicaid coverage even further. The states are statutorily given much latitude in structuring Medicaid benefits—already to the detriment of those who need treatment, but who rarely qualify (IOM, 1990). A reduction in Medicaid drug abuse treatment benefits would result in the shifting of patients from Medicaid to state agency and block grant funding (assuming those sources grow to meet the demand). Pharmaceutical companies are more favorably disposed to Medicaid financing than to direct public subsidies because Medicaid is an insurance mechanism (Rogowski, 1993). If Medicaid beneficiaries are shifted to private insurance by new subsidies for the purchase of private insurance, however, the pharmaceutical industry could benefit. Thus, the overall effect of reductions in Medicaid spending is uncertain. It will depend on the extent to which current Medicaid recipients purchase subsidized private insurance or are relegated to the public treatment system.

Additionally, the imposition of government price controls to reduce the costs of health care is inimical to the pharmaceutical industry. Price controls are seen as an unwarranted intrusion in the marketplace, and cutbacks in R&D spending have been threatened.

CONCLUSIONS

The most fundamental element of any health care reform—the extension of health insurance to at least some of the uninsured—can only have a beneficial effect on the development of anti-addiction medications. The inclusion of a prescription drug benefit also would encourage pharmaceutical development in general, but would not specifically guarantee investment in anti-addiction medications. The scope of drug abuse treatment benefits under any new legislation will have the most profound and direct effect on investment in anti-addiction medications. A pharmaceutical company contemplating investment will be more eager to proceed if the benefit does not impose arbitrary restrictions on treatment. A managed benefit that matches patients to the most appropriate care and a benefit that recognizes the commonalities between drug dependence and other chronic, relapsing medical conditions holds the greatest prospects for pharmaceutical investment. To remove the obstacle of uncertain or limited treatment financing, the federal government should consider providing adequate health insurance coverage for drug abuse treatment in a manner that is consistent with that for other chronic and relapsing medical conditions. Policies should be developed to provide for the matching of patients with the most effective treatment in the least restrictive setting.

REFERENCES

Arons BS, Frank RG, Goldman HH, McGuire TG, Stephens S. 1994. Mental health and substance abuse coverage under health reform. Health Affairs 13(1):192–205.

Batten H, Prottas J, Horgan CM, Simon LJ, Larson MJ, Elliott EA, Marsden ME. 1992. Drug Services Research Survey Final Report: Phase II. Waltham, MA: Bigel Institute for Health Policy, Brandeis University. Contract number 271-90-8319/1. Submitted to the National Institute of Drug Abuse, February 12, 1992.

CBO (Congressional Budget Office). 1994. How Health Care Reform Affects Pharmaceutical Research and Development. Washington, DC: CBO.

CRS (Congressional Research Service). 1994. Health Insurance. Washington, DC: Library of Congress, CRS. CRS Report No. IB 91093.

Harwood HJ, Thomsom M, Nesmith T. 1994. Healthcare Reform and Substance Abuse Treatment: The Cost of Financing Under Alternative Approaches. Fairfax, VA: Lewin-VHI.

IOM (Institute of Medicine). 1990. Treating Drug Problems. Gerstein DR and Harwood HJ, eds. Washington, DC: National Academy Press.

OTA (Office of Technology Assessment). 1993. Pharmaceutical R&D: Costs, Risks and Rewards. Washington, DC: U.S. Government Printing Office. OTA-H-522.

PMA (Pharmaceutical Manufacturers Association). 1993. Trends in U.S. Pharmaceutical Sales and R&D. Washington, DC: PMA.

Rogowski JA. 1993. Private Versus Public Sector Insurance Coverage for Drug Abuse. Santa Monica, CA: RAND Drug Policy Research Center. MR-166-DPRC.

Appendix H

Acronyms

AAPAA	American Academy of Psychiatrists in Alcoholism and Addiction
ABMS	American Board of Medical Specialties
ABPN	American Board of Psychiatry and Neurology
ACTH	adrenocorticotrophic hormone
ADAMHA	Alcohol, Drug Abuse, and Mental Health Administration
ADD	Antiepileptic Drug Development Program
ADEPT	Alcohol and Drug Education for Physician Training
AFDC	Aid to Families with Dependent Children
AIDS	acquired immune deficiency syndrome
ALS	amyotrophic lateral sclerosis (Lou Gehrig's disease)
AMBHA	American Managed Behavioral Healthcare Association
AMERSA	Association for Medical Education and Research in Substance Abuse
AMP	adenosine 3'5'-monophosphate
ASAM	American Society of Addiction Medicine
ATC	addiction training center
AZT	zidovudine
BDC	BioDevelopment Corporation
BJS	Bureau of Justice Statistics
BLS	Bureau of Labor Statistics
BSMD	Biobehavioral Sciences and Mental Disorders
CALDATA	California Drug and Alcohol Treatment Assessment
CASA	Center on Addiction and Substance Abuse
CBO	Congressional Budget Office

248

CDC	Centers for Disease Control and Prevention
CDDA	Commission on Medicines for Treatment of Drug Dependence and Abuse
CDER	Center for Drug Evaluation and Research
CDP	chemical dependency programs
CME	continuing medical education
CMHS	Center for Mental Health Services
CNS	central nervous system
CPDD	College on Problems of Drug Dependence
CRADAs	cooperative research and development agreements
CRS	Congressional Research Service
CSA	Controlled Substances Act
CSAP	Center for Substance Abuse Prevention
CSAT	Center for Substance Abuse Treatment
CTDP	Cocaine Treatment Discovery Program
DAWN	Drug Abuse Warning Network
DD	drug-discrimination test
DEA	Drug Enforcement Agency
DHHS	U.S. Department of Health and Human Services
DPC-PTR	Drug Price Competition and Patent Term Restoration Act
DSRS	Drug Services Research Survey
DVA	Department of Veterans Affairs
FDA	Food and Drug Administration
FDCA	Federal Food, Drug, and Cosmetic Act
FTEs	full-time equivalent personnel
FY	fiscal year
GAO	General Accounting Office
HIV	human immunodeficiency virus
HMO	health maintenance organization
HRSA	Health Resources and Services Administration
IDU	injecting drug-user
IND	investigational new drug
IOM	Institute of Medicine
IRB	institutional review board
K20	Scientist Development Award for Clinicians
K21	Scientist Development Award
LAAM	levo-alpha-acetylmethadol (trade name ORLAAM)
LMA	locomotor-activity test
LRP	Loan Repayment Program
MARC	Minority Access to Research Careers
MDD	Medications Development Division
MDMA	Methylenedioxymethamphetamine ("ecstacy")

MSH	melanocyte-stimulating hormone
NAS	National Academy of Sciences
NASADAD	National Association of State Alcohol and Drug Abuse Directors, Inc.
NATA	Narcotic Addict Treatment Act
NCDDG-AIDS	National Cooperative Drug Discovery Groups on Acquired Immune Deficiency Syndrome
NCI	National Cancer Institute
NCJA	National Criminal Justice Association
NDA	new drug application
NDATUS	National Drug and Alcoholism Treatment Survey
NIAAA	National Institute on Alcohol Abuse and Alcoholism Administration
NIAID	National Institute of Allergy and Infectious Diseases
NIDA	National Institute on Drug Abuse
NIH	National Institutes of Health
NRC	National Research Council
NRSA	National Research Service Awards
ODF	out-patient drug-free
ONDCP	Office of National Drug Control Policy
OPRR	Office of Protection from Research Risks
ORLAAM™	levo-alpha-acetylmethadol (LAAM)
OTA	Office of Technology Assessment
PBMs	pharmaceutical benefit managers
PCP	phencyclidine
PhRMA	Pharmaceutical Research and Manufacturers of America
PHS	Public Health Service
PMA	Pharmaceutical Manufacturers Association
POMC	pro-opiomelanocortin
R&D	research and development
R01	investigator-initiated grants
R18	research-demonstration grants
SA	self-administration test
SADAP	State Alcohol and Drug Abuse Profile
SAMHSA	Substance Abuse and Mental Health Services Administration
SSI	Supplemental Security Income
TB	tuberculosis
Tcs	therapeutic communities
TOPS	Treatment Outcome Prospective Study
TRUs	treatment research units
VA	Department of Veterans Affairs
WHO	World Health Organization